SOME ASSES JUST
NEED
WIPING

LESSONS ON HOLDING IT ALL TOGETHER
AS MY MOTHER'S LIFELONG CAREGIVER

SHELLY GRIMM

Some Asses Just Need Wiping
Lessons on Holding It All Together as My Mother's Lifelong Caregiver

Written by Shelly Grimm
Copyright © 2025 Peaceful Profits

Design and cover art by Peaceful Profits.

Paperback ISBN: 978-1-967587-40-7
eBook ISBN: 978-1-967587-41-4

This book is a work of nonfiction. It represents the accuracy of the events mentioned to the best of the author's recollection. Some names in the book have been replaced to maintain the privacy of certain individuals.

The information contained in this book is provided for educational purposes only and should not be construed as legal, financial, tax, or investment advice. Readers are strongly encouraged to consult with a qualified and licensed professional who can provide advice tailored to their individual circumstances. Laws, regulations, and financial practices vary across countries, states, and regions. Market conditions, returns, and outcomes will differ over time and cannot be guaranteed. While every effort has been made to provide accurate and timely information at the time of writing, we make no representations or warranties regarding completeness, accuracy, or applicability. We are not making any official legal or financial recommendations. The examples, figures, and principles presented herein are for illustrative and educational purposes only. Any decisions you make are solely your responsibility.

TABLE OF CONTENTS

DEDICATION

To my dear friend John,

This book is for you. You embody what it means to be a perpetual caregiver—a man whose courage, loyalty, and love have carried others through some of life's hardest battles. You have stood faithfully beside Tracy through her strokes, tending daily to her seizures and struggles with unwavering devotion. You have cared for your father through ALS, your brother through despair, your grandmother through her final years, and your mother as her constant support—all while raising two children on your own.

Many would have turned away, but you remain. Your bravery, compassion, and steadfastness shine as an extraordinary example of love in action.

John, whenever you doubt whether you are seen or heard, know this: You are. I admire you deeply, and I hope that whenever you open this book, you will be reminded of the profound impact your life and heart have on those around you.

Love ya!

INTRODUCTION

I touched down in New Orleans on July 10, 1982, feeling like I was starting a brand new chapter in my life. At 17 years old, I had only traveled out of my home state of Texas a few times, and those trips were by car to visit family. I felt like a real adult stepping out of the airplane. My boyfriend—a man ten years older than me who would later become my first husband—had just moved there. He was *gorgeous*, and I felt very special that he had paid for my flight just to spend the weekend together.

Little did I know that five months after my first visit, I would arrive in New Orleans for the last time as a visitor, and it would become my home for the next 39 years.

For the first time that I could remember, I felt liberated. You see, my mother, who had been a single parent since I was 3, had a chronic illness—Crohn's disease. She'd been in and out of hospitals throughout my entire childhood, and I'd been physically and emotionally caring for her for as long as I could remember. My trip to New Orleans felt like the beginning of a life of freedom. When I returned to Denton, Texas, after my trip to New Orleans, I'd be returning to my very own apartment. I was eager to start college at North Texas State University, now called the Univerity of North Texas, in a few weeks.

A day or two after my return, reality came crashing back in. My mother knocked on my apartment door for a "visit," which quickly became her move in. At the time, I was furious, and so was my dad. He was paying for the apartment and felt like it was just another instance of him caring for my mother, even though they'd been divorced for over a decade.

My boyfriend, Jimmy, continued to fly me out to New Orleans every other weekend, which provided some relief. Jimmy was a part owner of a health club where I worked in my hometown of Amarillo, and it was *not* love at first sight. I hated him at first. Now that I think about it, I should have held tight to that first impression. But who goes with their gut on something like that at age 16? Eventually, I fell for him—hard—ignoring every red flag along the way. Remember how I mentioned how *gorgeous* he was? I'm sure that had something to do with it.

During one of my visits, Jimmy shared that he'd been sexually abused by his father from about the age of 3 to 14. Instantly, my caregiver mode was activated. It was then that I was sure he NEEDED me! When I returned from that trip to Denton, filled with excitement about my newfound love, my new roommate—Mom—interpreted my teenage infatuation as mental illness. I learned later that those being cared for can become very territorial when it looks like their perpetual caregiver might flee. The feeling is even more profound if they feel their caregiver is being stolen from to care for someone else.

My mother had read a study indicating that manic depressive illness (now called bipolar I or II) is linked to high cortisol levels. She became so convinced this was what I was experiencing that she contacted a psychiatrist at the only local hospital in Denton. He recommended a series of blood tests to measure my cortisol levels. These blood tests had to be done multiple times a day for five days. The numerous blood draws throughout the day could only be done on an inpatient basis, and the only place that offered this was the local psychiatric unit.

So, for the better part of the second or third week of college, I attended college classes during the day and then slept in a mental ward to have blood drawn every four hours throughout the night. I had to stay in a special locked hospital room—not because I was a danger to myself or others, but because the staff wanted to protect me from some of the patients in the unit who were upset that I was allowed to leave during the day. I could hear the comments after I took my meds from the medication line: "Why is she special?"

The test results concluded that my cortisol levels were extremely high, likely indicating that they had been elevated for a long time. To medical professionals, this was no surprise, as the research showed that persistently high cortisol levels could be a sign of chronic, long-term stress. That explains a lot! I had been navigating one chaotic situation after another my entire life. But it didn't mean I was bipolar.

Don't get me wrong. I loved my mother dearly. She was my best friend. She was a fantastic person, and I learned so much from her, like keeping my sense of humor and surviving in this world no matter what life throws at me. Because of her illness, she wasn't a great parent, though. I parented myself *and* her throughout my childhood.

In a way, her lack of parenting skills made sense. When my mother first fell ill at the age of 18 in the late 1950s, she was initially diagnosed with terminal ileitis. When her doctor used the term "terminal", my mother naturally thought she had only a short time left on Earth. She never thought she would be the one to raise us, so she didn't strive for perfection in parenting. Instead, she was just trying to survive. Her condition was later renamed Crohn's disease, after Dr. Crohn. My mother had spent so many years believing she was on the verge of dying, only to realize that the classic definition of terminal no longer applied to her, and in reality, it never did. I wonder if their use of the word terminal in the very name of her initial diagnosis made an impression on how she perceived her condition at age 18?

But back to my brief stay in the mental hospital. They sent me home with a prescription for a daily sprinkle of lithium. I look back on that time today, and it all seems surreal, like it all happened to someone else. It was a very unusual experience, to say the least.

The stress level in my life was unlikely to change anytime soon. By that October, things had become too much in Denton. I quit school and moved to New Orleans to be with Jimmy. I gave him an ultimatum—a decision I deeply regret today—and we got married. Here I was, by God, in New Orleans. I planted my flag and was willing to die on that hill if I had to.

When I moved to New Orleans, many things started coming to light, as always. I was surprised to learn that Jimmy had already been married and divorced once before. His sister-in-law revealed this to me one day while I helped her prepare for a garage sale at her house. Later, when I was home alone, I found the divorce papers in his "important papers" box and discovered that his first wife divorced him due to psychological abuse. I was shocked! At the time of his first divorce, he was only 23.

I couldn't believe that someone so young could be so psychologically abusive to the extent that a young woman of the same age recognized it and took legal action! **You go, girl!!**

Ultimately, it wasn't long before I realized I had traded one burden for another, stepping back into a caregiving role I thought I had escaped. When I realized it, I felt like there was no way out. If I had only known that Jimmy didn't truly love me. I didn't know that given the type of abuse he'd experienced, he was potentially incapable of true love. It would take me many therapy sessions and reading books on the subject to understand why and heal from that bad decision.

Growing up as the child of someone with a chronic disease changed my life in ways that no child should have to endure. Over the years, many people—from family members to therapists—have wondered how I managed to get through it all without losing my mind or turning to addiction. As you'll see in the coming pages, the disease itself is what it is. My mother was in the fight for her very life every single day. I was along for the ride and had no choice in the matter. So it wasn't the disease itself that was to blame. It was all of the ancillary issues that came up along the way that were handled poorly or were left to a child who shouldn't have been making decisions. Sometimes, I question how I've come this far myself, but I did survive. I believe there is a reason for my survival, and I try to live that purpose out every day.

The Chronic Illness Epidemic

According to the American Medical Association (AMA), a chronic disease is a condition that lasts a year or more and requires ongoing medical care. These conditions can typically be managed but not cured. According to the World Health Organization (WHO), the Centers for Medicare & Medicaid Services (CMS), and the U.S. Department of Veterans Affairs (VA), chronic diseases often require daily medication.

So what does that mean? How significant is the problem of chronic illness in the United States today? As of 2024, three out of four adults had at least one chronic illness, and four out of ten had two or more.[1] The Centers for Disease Control (CDC) report that 51.4% of adults in the US suffer from multiple chronic conditions.[2] Additionally, 7 out of 10 people over the age of 65 will require care for some form of chronic illness before the end of their lives.[3]

These statistics are staggering, and for every patient represented in them, there is a caregiver (or several caregivers). We must change the conversations we're having around chronic illness and caregiving; as a society, we are already finding ourselves in

---

1   *Chronic Diseases in America*, Centers for Disease Control and Prevention, 2024, accessed February 22, 2025. https://www.cdc.gov/chronic-disease/about/index.html.

2   Peter Boersma and Tainya C. Clarke, "Multiple Chronic Conditions Among Adults Aged 18 and Over: United States, 2023." *Preventing Chronic Disease* 22 (2025): 240539. https://www.cdc.gov/pcd/issues/2025/24_0539.htm.

3   Melissa Favreault and Judith Dey. *What Is the Lifetime Risk of Needing and Receiving Long-Term Services and Supports?* Washington, DC: Office of the Assistant Secretary for Planning and Evaluation, U.S. Department of Health and Human Services, April 2016. https://aspe.hhs.gov/reports/what-lifetime-risk-needing-receiving-long-term-services-supports-0.

a very challenging situation. I cannot imagine what this might look like in 15 to 20 years.

It seems like everywhere I look, I'm greeted by smiling faces masking immense pain. Whether it be in the workplace, where I socialize, or on vacation—it almost doesn't seem to matter where I find myself—those smiling faces are all around me. My question remains: Is it just me? Am I able to see them because I'm one of them? Or are there just so many hurting caregivers out there?

The Story Behind This Book

In this book, I will talk about the impact of chronic illness on families from my perspective as a caregiver during my childhood and early adult years. I will tell some of my personal stories and tell it like it was—no sugarcoating or tiptoeing around the truth. And don't worry, we'll have some fun along the way too. My stories are full of humor and humanity. For each one, I'll point out how things could have turned out differently had the people around me made different choices about how to support me better.

This book talks about the hidden symptoms of chronic illness. There's a lot of dysfunction that most people don't recognize behind the scenes. When a child becomes the caregiver, they become the parent (if they are capable), and the parent becomes the child (or at least assumes that role emotionally). I know because that was my life. I hope that my story can help shed light on the ways we, as a society and as individuals, can help prevent children of chronically ill parents from slipping through the cracks like I did.

How It Started

At 18 years of age, my mother became the first known female case of Crohn's disease in the United States. I spent my childhood caring for her. Then, I lived my early adult years in a severely dysfunctional relationship with a mentally ill husband. My firstborn child, my son Ben, was born on the spectrum before the spectrum even existed, and I was a single mother to both my boys while again caring for my mother until her death. Today, I'm married to a wonderful man who happens to have Kawasaki disease, for which he'll be on medication for the rest of his life.

My entire life has revolved around chronic illness, and it's been both a blessing and a curse. I learned to be strong and take care of myself. Because I was so capable, no one ever felt that I was in any danger. Some parts of my life appeared relatively normal. For example, we ate dinner at my grandmother's house nearly every night when my mother had the energy to drive... but that was mainly because there was rarely any food in our refrigerator.

There were good times too, like Saturdays when my father picked me up to go "rat killing," and the times I spent down the street at my friend Cindy's house. The times her grandmother took us to her house in Plainview during the summer were also great. We'd spend a week there with no air conditioning, sleeping with the windows wide open, and sweating our brains out. Cindy also had a mother with medical issues, so we both took on a lot of responsibilities at home. I look back on that friendship now as a lifesaver, and we are still in touch today.

Chronic illness has a devastating, long-lasting effect on children and family members, especially if the chronically ill person is a parent or primary breadwinner of the family. The impact of chronic illness goes much deeper than the toll a long-term physical illness takes because it affects relationships at a deep level. If support systems for the caregivers and the ill family member are not identified and established early on, the caregiver's relationships may become permanently dysfunctional and last for generations.

This book is my way of focusing on the blessings while helping others avoid the pitfalls of caregiver roles. It will help you look closer at those who care for the chronically ill people around you. It will also cause you to examine yourself and see how you can become part of the solution or find better support when you enter caregiver roles.

Look at the statistics about chronic illness in the introduction again. The numbers are staggering, and it seems like a chronic illness attacks our friends and family members around every corner. It would be easy to become numb or desensitized to the number of people who suffer from chronic illnesses and to stop seeing them. But we can't turn a blind eye to the children affected by chronic diseases within their families. And we definitely can't stop showing compassion for the caregivers.

Because someday, we are the ones who might need care.

Who This Book is For

I've written this book for women who care for children with special needs, parents with chronic illnesses, or both. Many find themselves in the "sandwich generation" caring for children and aging parents or close relatives simultaneously. If that describes you, let me formally introduce myself.

Hi, my name is Shelly Grimm. I have been in the financial services industry since 1997. This book will explore the experiences that sparked my passion for this profession. Every day, I help people navigate their protection needs and create plans to avoid placing their loved ones in tenuous financial situations due to chronic illness and unexpected loss. I'm also a huge advocate for the children and caregivers impacted by chronically ill family members.

When you finish this book, you will know how to better support children affected by a family member's chronic illness. You will learn how to better protect and prepare these children and how to recognize those who are struggling, which can lead to meaningful conversations about how you can help.

At the end of our time together, I hope you'll better understand that even unseen chronic illnesses—like many autoimmune diseases—are just as devastating as diseases that cause openly identifiable conditions where the patient wears their wound or disease openly, like an amputated leg or arm.

This book will also expose the ways chronic illness can dominate a family and cause dysfunctional generational patterns around caregiving if not handled correctly.

In the first half of this book, I take you behind the scenes of my childhood, from ages 5 to 13. I peel it back to the beginning, to the things no 5-year-old should ever have to deal with. Along the way, I'll show you how things could have gone differently in hopes that this perspective can keep what happened to me from happening to another child.

In the book's second half, I bring this introduction full circle. You'll follow me from age 13, when I became legally emancipated and lived by myself, to age 17, when I left my hometown to marry a narcissistic abuser. As I said, I went from one caregiving situation to another, and I never even saw it coming.

When caregiving begins at a young age and children are praised for doing a great job or making the patient feel better, it can create a lasting pattern in their lives. Adult children often find it challenging to recognize that the world outside their loved ones is different. While others may readily accept our help, they might be slow or completely unwilling to reciprocate with the same level of compassion or care. Nowadays, everyone is facing their issues to some degree. Caregivers tend to neglect their needs because they have been conditioned to believe that the patient or person in need comes first, with caregivers often placing themselves last. I spent decades overexerting myself, trying to help and please everyone around me.

We can't remain healthy as individuals, families, or societies unless we collectively gather to first care for ourselves. Our society's approach to dealing with chronic illness has been broken for far too long. It didn't take a day to get here, and it will take longer than a day to get out, but we have to start somewhere.

I've compiled some valuable resources at the end of each chapter. If you're feeling uncertain about your organizational and legacy planning and want to discuss that, I've provided a way for you to connect with me online in the resources section in the back of this book.

Thanks for being here and taking this journey with me.

Shelly Grimm

WHAT QUALIFIES AS A CHRONIC ILLNESS?

The most common chronic illnesses in the United States include:

Cardiovascular Diseases
Hypertension (High Blood Pressure), Coronary Artery Disease (CAD), Congestive Heart Failure (CHF), Stroke, Peripheral Artery Disease (PAD)

Metabolic and Endocrine Disorders
Diabetes (Type 1 and Type 2), Hypothyroidism, Hyperthyroidism, Polycystic Ovary Syndrome (PCOS), Metabolic Syndrome

Respiratory Diseases
Chronic Obstructive Pulmonary Disease (COPD), Asthma, Cystic Fibrosis, Pulmonary Hypertension

Autoimmune and Inflammatory Diseases
Rheumatoid Arthritis, Lupus (Systemic Lupus Erythematosus), Multiple Sclerosis (MS), Crohn's Disease, Ulcerative Colitis, Psoriasis/Psoriatic Arthritis

Neurological Disorders
Alzheimer's Disease, Parkinson's Disease, Epilepsy, Migraines and Chronic Headaches

Chronic Pain Conditions
Fibromyalgia, Chronic Fatigue Syndrome (Myalgic Encephalomyelitis), Osteoarthritis, Complex Regional Pain Syndrome (CRPS)

Gastrointestinal Disorders
Irritable Bowel Syndrome (IBS), Gastroesophageal Reflux Disease (GERD), Celiac Disease, Chronic Liver Disease (Cirrhosis, Fatty Liver Disease)

Mental Health and Psychiatric Disorders
Major Depressive Disorder, Generalized Anxiety Disorder, Bipolar Disorder, Schizophrenia, Post-Traumatic Stress Disorder (PTSD)

Chronic Infectious Diseases
HIV/AIDS, Hepatitis B & C, Tuberculosis (latent or active)

Other Chronic Conditions
Chronic Kidney Disease (CKD), Sickle Cell Disease, Osteoporosis, Obesity (as a chronic condition)

PART 1

Parenting My Parent

Chapter 1

Going to the Hospital

T he earliest memory I have of my mother being ill is the day my grandmother brought me to the High Plains Baptist Hospital to say goodbye to her. I was only 5-years-old at the time, but her health problems had started years before that when she was just 18. She fell critically ill on the way home from her senior trip to San Antonio. Instead of returning to Amarillo High School to meet the parents, the driver went straight to St. Anthony's Hospital. This hospital was better known for being the hospital for women and children in our small town.

Upon arrival, they took her symptoms to indicate she was having a female medical complication. They rushed her to surgery and when they opened her up, they found that her small intestine was completely blocked due to swelling. They resected a large portion of her small bowel and closed her up. She was eventually diagnosed with terminal ileitis, becoming the first female ever documented with this condition in the United States and one of only five cases nationwide. When my older sister was born a few years later, my mother became the first woman to have a baby with active terminal ileitis. As you can imagine, the medical community wasn't sure what to do with her.

Because there were so few other cases, and none of them were women, what they knew about the disease and how to treat it was minimal. To make matters even more complicated, the only other people in the nation with this diagnosis were four Jewish men. This led physicians and scientists to believe the condition only affected those of Middle Eastern descent. It's not like they could just open a medical journal and read all about it. It was just too new. Doctors and surgeons treated her the best they could as they worked to learn more. The initial treatment was surgery and then heavy doses of prednisone to reduce the swelling and inflammation.

Today, we know this disease as Crohn's disease—a type of inflammatory bowel disease (IBD) that causes swelling and irritation of the digestive tract tissue. Symptoms include belly pain, severe diarrhea, fatigue, weight loss, and malnutrition.[4] Sounds like a really fun party, right? We are no closer to a cure today than we were back then, and Crohn's remains a painful, debilitating disease that can lead to serious or life-threatening complications. My mother fought Crohn's disease for 47 years before she finally succumbed to it at the age of 64.

If she had been an 18-year-old diagnosed with Crohn's disease today, she'd have access to all sorts of treatment options. With the proper care, she could have even gone into long-term remission and lived a more functional life…but that's not

---

4   Mayo Clinic Staff. "Inflammatory Bowel Disease (IBD)." *Mayo Clinic*, last modified April 19, 2024. https://www.mayoclinic.org/diseases-conditions/inflammatory-bowel-disease/symptoms-causes/syc-20353315

her story. And because of that, my story starts as a 5-year-old walking into a hospital with no idea that her life was about to become a really wild ride.

High Plains Baptist Hospital

I knew my mom had been sick, but I wasn't aware of how ill she really was. We had just returned from Oklahoma City, where we'd been staying at my grandmother's house. Mother had a bad flare-up, so we'd all come back to Amarillo, my grandmother included. That's where her ileitis doctors practiced. Surgeons at High Plains Baptist Hospital had performed a resection—the surgical removal of a damaged or diseased part of the body—of her small intestine. Unfortunately, she had become septic and was no longer responding to the antibiotics. The doctors had shared with my grandmother that short of a miracle from God, my mother would not be leaving the hospital this time.

But I didn't know any of that as my grandmother, my sister Tanya, and I entered High Plains Baptist Hospital that day.

The hospital wouldn't let anyone under 14 onto the upper floors where the patient rooms were, so we all went to the main waiting room. The big room looked gigantic to this tiny 5-year-old, and it was empty except for the three of us.

Ding. My head swiveled towards the sound as the elevator doors slid open.

And there she was—my mommy! The nurses wheeled her in, complete with the hospital bed, IVs, heart monitor and all, out of the elevator and over to where we were sitting. As the nurses set the brake on the hospital bed, my grandmother picked me up and placed me next to the most important person in my life, the only one I had ever lived with. She looked so weak, frail, and sick—I was trembling all over. Her voice was barely a whisper as she asked everyone around us to give us a few moments alone.

I wasn't sure what that meant. I thought we were there to visit with everyone. Then my mom opened her mouth and started to speak.

"Michelle, Mommy's really sick," she said. Back then, I was still Michelle. No one called me Shelly until I was a little older. "I don't think I'm going to be coming home. This might be the last time you see me. You'll probably be going to live with your dad. Grandmother will be around, and so will Tanya, so you'll still see everyone."

I don't remember another word that was said, but I remember crying. What was my mom saying? How could it be that I'd never see her again? I *never* wanted not to see her again! I didn't want to live with my dad. My world was rocked, and my 5-year-old brain couldn't understand what was happening.

When we finished talking, the nurses wheeled the hospital bed—and my mommy—back into the elevator. My grandmother followed them, saying, "I'll be right back." The doors closed behind them, leaving me with my sister in the waiting room. I sat in that waiting room, 5 years old, wondering what I'd do next. My 13-year-old sister did not comfort or reassure me that things would be all right. Even she wasn't sure things were going to be okay.

From that day forward, my life felt uncertain and unstable, and things would never be the same.

I've asked myself over and over through the years what kind of world we live in that it's acceptable to tell a 5-year-old, "Your mother's dying," and then all the adults leave the room. Think about it—everyone followed the person who was dying, but no one stayed with the children who were going to live. It was traumatic.

Although my mother lived, I spent the rest of her life knowing the inevitable was coming and waiting for the day when she'd be gone.

I wasn't the only child in my family who had this experience. When my sister was 9 or 10, our grandmother drove her down to Temple, Texas, where mom was in the hospital, to "say goodbye." But even though we had the same mother and shared some of the same experiences, the ways we handled life with her chronic illness were very different. I don't know if it was the eight-year age gap, but honestly, I don't even think we lived in the same reality when it came to our mother.

My mother's illness shaped my life; it was a constant presence. I learned early on that Crohn's disease didn't just affect her body—it impacted our entire lives. A hospital stay, a financial crisis, or a new complication always required me to step up, and I did so even from a very young age. A 5-year-old should never be left to feel like they are carrying the entire world on their shoulders. But that's how I felt

My sister couldn't handle it. She left as soon as possible, moving in with our grandmother instead of staying with our mom and me. Grandmother alway stayed around long enough for Mother to get back on her feet, then she'd return to Oklahoma. I remember when my sister called our grandmother and asked her to come and get her. She was done. The house had no food, and she wasn't about to stick around any longer waiting for it to magically appear. I don't even really blame her. She saw a way out and took it.

My grandmother drove four hours from Oklahoma City to pick her up. When she pulled up, my sister grabbed her things and left—just like that, without a second thought, regret, or looking back. And me? Well, of course, I stayed.

Nobody asked if I wanted to go, either. I don't think they even considered it. I don't know if they thought I was fine, if they thought we'd figure it out, or if they just didn't think about me at all. But I do know this—when that car drove away, I was still there, in a house with no food, a sick mother, and no choice but to deal with it.

My sister never really physically took care of our mother. When she was little, they lived with my grandmother most of the time. When my mom married my father, my sister still wanted to live with my grandmother, and for the most part, she did. I have always believed that is why she saw things so differently.

Even as adults, my sister and I handled things very differently. In 1986, my mother moved to Oklahoma City to live with my sister. She'd been living with my then-husband Jimmy, and me, but Jimmy had grown tired of being second to my mother and her meddling, so he wanted her to leave. My mother stayed with Tanya for about six months, but things took a turn for the worse. Mom called and asked me to come and get her because Tanya was "throwing her out." I agreed to fly up there and drive her and her belongings back to New Orleans.

My sister called as soon as I'd hung up with my mother. She told me to "just leave her." She said, "Let her figure it out. This isn't your problem. She's never been forced to stand on her own two feet!"

But how could I do that? How could I just ignore her requests for help? That was our mother. I couldn't turn my back on her. That just wasn't in me.

The thing is, I don't think my sister was being cruel. She just couldn't deal with it. She was protecting herself, drawing lines where I never could. Maybe she thought I was weak for always saying yes. Perhaps she thought she was strong enough to say no. Her husband helped a lot by refusing to let my mother interfere with their lives after that. My mother wrote to my sister for two years, trying to speak with her. My brother-in-law read the letters as they came and tore them up if he didn't think they would benefit my sister. Sometimes, I wonder how many of those letters she ever even saw.

If She Had Stayed

When it comes to coping with a family member's chronic illness, it's not easy for anyone involved. If you're an adult caregiver or someone with a chronic disease and there are children in your life who are impacted—and they are *always* impacted—there's an opportunity for you to do things differently so that you can protect those children. I don't think anyone today would agree that it's okay to leave a 5-year-old on their own in a hospital waiting room after they have just received the worst news of their life. Yet that's what happened to me, and I don't want any other child to experience something like that.

There were countless opportunities throughout my childhood that, had anyone stepped in, could have made a massive difference in my life. One such opportunity was that day I sat in the hospital waiting room after being told my mother was dying. What if someone had stepped in, even in a small way? I'd like to reimagine the scene with another outcome so you can see how things might have turned out differently.

Back then, nobody could figure out what to do with me. Even on what everyone thought was her deathbed, my mom was saying, "Well, you'll probably live with your dad. Maybe." I was handed the kind of uncertainty that no 5-year-old can deal with. Let's stop and rewind to right there, the point where the nurses start pushing my mom's hospital bed back to the elevators.

Imagine if my grandmother had stayed with me instead of leaving me alone in the waiting room and following the nurses back to my mother's hospital room. What if she had sat down in one of those uncomfortable chairs with me and seen me? First, you would have had to provide me with a different grandmother for that, but while we are imagining things, let's go big!

"It's gonna be all right," she could have said. "Nothing's gonna happen to you. We've got you. You've got your daddy, you've got your big sister, and you've got me. You've got all kinds of people who are going to help you. We'll take care of you and make sure you're okay."

Wouldn't that have created a better result for that little 5-year-old learning that her mother is dying and letting that be the only thing she heard that day?

Remember the Shelly you met in the introduction? The girl who stepped off a plane in New Orleans into what she thought was freedom on July 10, 1982? If 5-year-old Michelle had been supported that day in the hospital waiting room—if she had known beyond a shadow of a doubt that she had people who would care for her instead of her feeling like she had to carry the weight of caregiving as a child—wouldn't things have turned out differently on July 10, 1982?

I was a 17-year-old girl flying to New Orleans to see an older boyfriend she definitely shouldn't even be seeing, but it sounded fun, and he was a hunk.

Nobody was looking out for me or pointing out red flags. How could they? I was the one parenting my parents. They couldn't expect me to act like a parent and then try to parent me. But what if someone had parented me? If that scene at the hospital when I was 5 had been set differently, how would my life have changed?

The Critical Truth

Millions upon millions of people are dealing with one or more chronic illnesses in the United States right now, and it's not just the person with the disease who's affected. Don't forget about the caregivers, especially the children who have fallen into the caregiving role, like I did. If you haven't already, I invite you to open your eyes.

Maybe you're a caregiver yourself. If so, use the lessons you learn in this book to help those in your circle know how to help you.

Maybe you're the one struggling with a chronic illness yourself. If so, use the lessons in this book to ensure you're helping your family members, especially the children, feel supported and cared for. You want them to make it out of childhood without ending up selling drugs or turning tricks on a street corner, right?

As soon as a caregiver is needed, action must be taken, especially if that caregiver is a child. Even a seemingly small action can make a massive difference for a child of someone with a chronic illness, especially if they're in a caregiver role. Here are a few examples to get you started:

- Speaking a kind word.
- Offering transportation.
- Dropping off groceries.
- Attending their school events when their ill parent can't.
- Inviting them over for a meal and allowing them to just play.
- Talking to their teachers to make sure they're aware of the situation.
- Being their pen pal.

- Sponsoring their shoes or gear for an extracurricular activity they love.

There are a million different ways to show support to a caregiver, adult *or* child. Pick one. Or not, it's up to you. But I hope you will act. No matter how mature a child seems, they're still a child. They still need someone to have their back.

I was the mature kid everyone assumed was doing okay. "Oh, that's just Michelle. She'll be fine." Inside, however, I was drowning.

I'm not bitter today, but my inner 5-year-old child still grieves. I'm heartbroken at the thought of the other 5-year-old children out there who are going through this. They shouldn't have to, at least not alone. Every step could have been different for me had anybody done anything different from age 5 to July 10, 1982. This chapter is just one example, and you'll read many more throughout the rest of this book.

So, where was my dad in all of this? In the next chapter, I will tell you what was going on with the other side of my family. Stick around because it reads like a fairytale—but not the good kind. I'm talking about evil stepmother-type stuff.

Chapter 2

Life Goes On

L ife didn't pause just because my mother almost died. Nobody gave me even a single moment to breathe. No one sat me down and said, "Hey, kid, that was scary, huh? Let's talk about it." It didn't work like that for me.

Mom finally left the hospital, and I became the sweet little girl who took care of things.

It hadn't always been that way. By the time Mom had her hospital stay when I was 5, she had been sick for ten years. I was just too young to realize it until then. After my parents divorced when I was 3, we moved into a house my dad gave my mother in the divorce on Clifton Street.

My mom was a copywriter and had begun working at McCann Advertising in Amarillo. It wasn't long before we all moved to Oklahoma City, and my mom was offered a copywriter's position in the Oklahoma City office of McCann Advertising. My earliest fond memories are of living in Oklahoma City, and I loved it there. I still remember the playground near our apartment and going to preschool and kindergarten nearby.

We ended up back in Texas only for that life-changing hospital stay because my mom got sick again, and this time, it was terrible. Crohn's disease was still so new that doctors in Oklahoma City didn't know how to treat her illness, so we went back to Texas and the doctors who had diagnosed her. We pretty much drove straight to the hospital. My sister was already staying with my grandmother when we returned. I went to stay at my dad's. Even after Mom left the hospital, my sister never really lived with us full-time again. She was 13 by then and stayed in our childhood home only when it was more convenient for her for school or whatnot.

When my mother left the hospital, we moved back into the house on Clifton that my dad had given her in the divorce. Grandmother stayed with us for a few days until Mom regained some of her strength. Even after that, it was a long time before she had the strength to walk up the one big step from the sidewalk to the porch. Around the six-month mark, I remember having to go next door and ask a neighbor to help me get her inside once because she physically couldn't lift herself a single step.

She may have helped take care of things after Mom's hospitalization, but that doesn't mean Grandmother was a warm or comforting person. She and I had a good relationship, but she wasn't the kind of woman who held your hand and told you everything would be okay. She had lived through some of the most challenging times in history, including the Dust Bowl and the Depression. It made her practical and tough as nails. She was there to do what needed to be done—and make no mistake, she was dependable and steady as they come—but she was not there to offer hugs or soothing words.

My mother used to tell me that the reason she didn't die in that hospital when I was 5 was because of me. For a long time, I believed her. I believed she kept fighting because she loved me so much, and there was nowhere else for me to go. But now that I've lived a little and looked back with clearer eyes, I don't think that was the entire reason.

Teena Ridge—my mother—didn't want to be invisible. She didn't want to be written off, put away, or pitied. She needed to be useful. She needed a purpose, so she made herself the martyr and told herself, "I'm doing this for Michelle." But it wasn't just about me. It was about holding on to something that made her feel like she still had value in a world that doesn't know what to do with sick women in their 20s and 30s.

When chronic illness or disability enters a relationship, the balance shifts—sometimes slowly, sometimes all at once—but it constantly shifts. The roles that once felt equal begin to tilt. When the roles that should have been weighted more towards a parent's shift to the child, like what happened with my mother and me, the difference in balance can feel enormous.

This dynamic is difficult enough for two adults to manage. The shared weight of the world starts to lean a little more to one side, and eventually, one partner finds themselves carrying more than they ever expected. That's what happened to a good friend of mine and her husband. They used to be incredibly active—skiing, golfing, always on the move. Their relationship was built on doing life side by side. But four years into their marriage, my friend experienced a series of strokes, and everything changed. Suddenly, her husband wasn't just her husband anymore—he became her caregiver, advocate, and full-time support system. It was a very difficult adjustment for them.

And the most challenging part? It's not just the physical strain. It's the emotional shift that happens when love has to stretch to include assistance, appointments, and the quiet ache of watching someone you love lose pieces of their independence. It's hard, and I learned young that nobody would make me feel safe. Nobody would scoop me up and tell me that things were okay. Life moved on, whether I was ready or not.

My Mother, The Duchess

That's not to say there weren't people nearby who *wanted* to help my mother. I remember the lady next door. Her name was Linda. Bless her heart, and she really did want to help. But my mother wasn't the kind of person who just *took* help. Oh, no. She had particular rules about *how* she would receive it, *when* it could be offered, and *on what terms* the help would be accepted. And if you didn't meet those conditions or she found you annoying or disliked you, your good intentions were dead on arrival.

And trust me, my mother did not even try to mask the fact that she was annoyed with you for being there in her presence when she didn't ask for or want to receive your version of help. She could tell a person to go pound sand without even a smile on her face or a pleasant tone in her voice, making it sound polite. She preferred the direct, bitchy method so that you never returned with an offer of help ever again.

My mother wanted to run her ship, even if it sank. And when she was on steroids, which were often prescribed for her flare-ups, you never knew who you were gonna get. One day, she'd be all smiles, chatting away like she enjoyed your presence, and the next, you'd swear she was a completely different person—irritated, snappy, ready to send you right back out the door you walked in.

That was just how she was. You didn't just *do* something for her. You did it *her way*, when *she* decided, and only on *her* terms. And if you didn't? You were dismissed. No exceptions. And if that sounds like the behavior of someone who grew up thinking the world revolved around them…well, you wouldn't be wrong.

My mother hadn't always been sick. She wasn't always the frail woman lying in bed, dictating orders between bites of baby food. No, once upon a time, my mother, Teena, was the Duchess. That's what my grandfather called her, and it wasn't just some cute nickname. She *earned* it. The first six years of her life, she was an only child, fitting the definition of a spoiled kid to a T.

Like I said, my grandmother was not the doting, affectionate type. During the 1930s, life wasn't just hard—it was barely survivable. She was the oldest of six siblings, raising her two kids while taking care of her widowed mother and trying to scrape together some semblance of a life in a place where crops wouldn't grow and there was barely enough to eat.

My grandfather had helped build the Hoover Dam and had worked on other Teddy Roosevelt infrastructure projects across the United States until those ran out. Then, the family settled in Amarillo, where he worked for the railroad. He always wanted to be a conductor, but he was colorblind, so an engineer was as high as he could go. Meanwhile, my grandmother ran a household with more people than she preferred and not enough hands.

Then, there was Teenie.

The child who had been born into all of this and somehow still managed to be the show's star. My grandfather doted on her, spoiling her with attention, while my grandmother…well, let's just say she had no time for nonsense.

Teena liked to push limits and test boundaries. She had this habit of getting into things she had no business getting into, and my grandmother didn't have the patience for it. There's a story that says everything about my mother, grandmother, and the kind of family we came from.

One day, my grandfather came home from work to find Teena tied to a tree in the front yard, her hands bound behind her back.

"What are you doing out here?" he asked.

My mother, 8 years old and completely unbothered, shrugged. "Mother tied me up."

I don't know what my mother had done—probably something she'd been told not to do at least a dozen times—but I know my grandmother. She wasn't threatening to discipline her child. She followed through. And on that particular day, tying Teenie to a tree must have seemed like the most efficient way to deal with her.

My grandfather shook his head, sighed, and told her, "Well, let me go inside and see if I can untie you."

He went into the house, returned a few minutes later, and said, "Nope. I can't. But here's some water."

And that was that.

If that sounds harsh, remember—this was the 1940s in the Texas Panhandle. Parenting wasn't gentle. Life wasn't gentle. There were no books on how to raise a strong-willed, high-maintenance child. You just did what you had to do. And if tying your daughter to a tree was what it took to get a moment of peace, then that's what you did.

And Teenie? She discovered that she had to fight for what she wanted and demand control over the people around her. Teenie also realized that if she wanted something, she had to dictate exactly how she expected it to happen, but she would have to fight against her strong-willed mother, who was determined to put her in her place.

And that never changed.

So, no, my mother wasn't just some sick woman who got cranky when people tried to help. She had always been that way. She had *always* wanted things her way or not at all.

And if you didn't fall in line?

You could hit the road, Jack!

Almost Remarried...Again

You're probably wondering where my father was in all of this. I had stayed with him a lot while Mother was in the hospital. He had his own very successful business, and since he wasn't punching a time clock like other dads, he had the flexibility to take me to nursery school when Mom was too sick to get out of bed. So what happened to that kind of help after she made her recovery? Well, it's complicated.

After Grandmother had gone home, my dad came around a lot, checking in on her and me. He'd pick me up from school and drop me off, bring food by, and help in other ways he knew how. It must have started to feel familiar, comfortable, and maybe even redemptive at some point. I didn't realize it back then, but during that time, my parents almost got remarried for a third time. They even scheduled an appointment with the justice of the peace.

But on the wedding morning, my dad woke up with a moment of clarity—or panic. Maybe both. He called my mom and said, "It didn't work the first time. It didn't work the second time. What on earth makes us think the third time's the charm?"

And that was that. The wedding was off. As far as I know, there was no fight or big dramatic meltdown. Just two people—who did, in their own messy, wounded way, love each other—realizing that love wouldn't be enough. Even my mom later said she didn't know what they were thinking. I think, deep down, they both knew the truth. None of the problems we had, including my mother's illness, were going to magically go away just because they said "I do" again. They loved each other, but would never make it work in this lifetime.

I know my father loved me in his way, but there were no fatherly, "I've got you, kid" moments. Except for maybe when my mother was in the hospital on her deathbed, living with my dad was never even a serious conversation. His house wasn't a safe haven either, and I'll explain why later in this chapter.

There was also the fact that even at a very young age, my presence comforted my mother. Even if it would have been better for me to live with someone else, she refused to be separated from me. I was an easygoing child who never thought to question why I lived where I lived. I accepted the way things were without question, maybe because underneath it all, even at 5 years old, I understood there was nowhere in the world that was truly safe for me. Not Mom's house, not Grandmother's house, and definitely not Daddy's house. I had to figure things out on my own.

My Father, King of the Castle

My dad was born in 1927, right before the Great Depression hit. During his childhood, the Texas Panhandle was nothing but dust and despair. The Dust Bowl didn't just strip the land bare—it made people hard. It made them do whatever it took to survive, and my father was no exception.

He was sent away at a young age to a Catholic military boarding school up in St. Paul, Minnesota. My uncle was sent there too, but he hated it and left as soon as possible. My father, though, thrived in the structure. He loved the rules, the discipline, and the order of it all. It gave him a sense of control over a world that, at home, had seemed like nothing but chaos. After school, he went straight into the Navy, served in World War II, and then came home and went to Texas A&M, where he fit right in with the regimented, no-nonsense culture of the Corps of Cadets.

That was my father—precise, disciplined, and structured. He wasn't the type to give big speeches or throw his arms around you in a bear hug. He was a man of quiet responsibility who showed his love by doing rather than saying. He was always physically present in my life, but never really emotionally available.

It wasn't that he didn't love me—I never doubted that he did. But he loved me in the only way he knew how. Through consistency. Through ritual. Through small, reliable gestures that were his version of saying I mattered to him.

Rat Killing and Ice Cream With Daddy

Daddy and I had some of the best days together from ages 5 to 7 in those early years. Every Saturday morning, he'd pick me up, and we'd go "rat killing." Now, we weren't hunting rats— that was his term for running errands, checking on things, tidying up loose ends. But it meant one crucial thing: I got to spend time with my dad.

The first stop was always his print shop. My father was a successful and influential man who owned several printing-related businesses—print shops, printing supply companies, and paper companies, among others. In the '70s and '80s, he employed more employees than most other businesses in the area. And every Saturday morning, he'd pick me up and take me with him to wrap up whatever work needed to be finished from the week. I'd wander around the shop, soaking in the smell of ink and paper, watching as the presses ran and his employees bustled around.

They all knew me there. They'd humor me by making little printing plates with my name on them and rolling out fresh copies of whatever I wanted. Every Saturday, I felt like I was part of something for a few hours. They always used the excess paper from their jobs to make notepads to use around the office. For me, they'd run out a batch with my name proudly displayed at the top. I never left without a stack of personalized notepads, and it made me feel very special.

After we wrapped up at the shop, we'd head over to another business my dad owned with my uncle—Graphic, Equipment & Supply, a printing equipment and parts distribution sales business. My dad and uncle would sit and talk shop over lunch, and I'd listen to their conversations, half bored, half fascinated. The bill was always a battle between them. They had this unspoken game where whoever grabbed the check first had to pay. And let me tell you, neither of them ever wanted to be the one to grab it first.

I'd watch them sit there, talking, waiting each other out, and neither one reaching for the check. I'd stretch out in the booth, sometimes even doze off, while they stubbornly refused to be the first to give in. Eventually, they'd run out of things to say. One of them would sigh, shake his head, and say, "Well, I guess I'm paying then," and finally reach for it. The other would smirk in victory.

To me, those Saturdays were the best days.

Then there were Sunday nights. No matter what was going on or how busy he was, my dad would pick me up and take me to get ice cream every Sunday night. Sometimes it was Dairy Queen, sometimes Baskin-Robbins, but it didn't matter where we went. It was about the ritual. I could count on that time with him. It was ours.

When my birthday rolled around in November, Baskin-Robbins would send out their little coupon—you better believe we cashed that in *immediately*. It didn't matter if it was one or two weeks early. If my dad got that coupon in the mail, he'd pick me up regardless of what day of the week it was and say, "Let's go get your birthday ice cream."

That was how my dad loved me—through little things that most people might not even notice, but that meant the world to me. And I think it meant the world to him, too, because he called me his crown jewel on his deathbed to both of my boys when they had their last conversations with him.

Why I Couldn't Live at the Castle

But despite all of that, despite how much I loved those Saturday mornings and Sunday nights, I couldn't live with him. It wasn't even a question. My brother lived there, and my brother...well, he had problems.

My father had been married to another woman before my mother and had a son—my half brother—who was in his custody. My brother was nine years older than I was, and he was angry and volatile. The guy was a fury-filled storm just waiting to happen.

He wasn't always cruel to me, but he *was* unpredictable, which made me fearful. He could be playful one moment, if you want to call tickling me until I cried playful, and terrifying the next. When I was 3 years old, he got angry with me for playing with his lawn darts, so he tied me to a tree and threw darts at me. When my dad came home and found me tied to a tree, you better believe my big brother was in big trouble.

He didn't just have problems at home, either. By age 5, he'd been banned from riding the school bus for misbehavior. By the time I was 5 and he was 14, he had already been kicked out of more boarding schools than I could count. My dad didn't know how to handle him, so he sent him away to every program he could find, but nothing stuck. My brother would get kicked out, come home, wreak havoc, and the cycle would start again.

That house was never peaceful, but it's possible that I could have spent more time there when my brother was away. Things were fantastic when it was just my dad and me. But something was about to happen that would change all that. My father got remarried. I'll tell you more about that in chapter 4, but that added another layer to the craziness that was my life. Even sadder was the fact that there were few resources available to a little girl like me in the '60s and '70s.

Caring Without a Net

Back in the 1960s and 1970s, when someone got sick—especially someone like my mom—it wasn't a matter of *how* we were going to care for her. It was just assumed we would, no questions asked. That's how things were done. Families took care of their own.

Unless you were ultra-wealthy, there were no private nurses or full-time caregivers. No coordinated care teams or home health aides showed up to check vitals and chart progress. And even if there had been, we weren't that kind of family. If someone was sick or disabled, your people took care of you. Period. You didn't *get* help—you *were* the help.

Not only that, but for my mother, the idea of being "on assistance" was worse than being sick. We begged her to stay on state aid when she was at her lowest. Back then, before Social Security Disability even existed, the only thing available was Medicaid, and you had to petition your congressman to get help. It was a welfare system, plain and simple. It had no dignity—at least not in how it was presented.

Even though she was qualified—even though she *needed* it—every time my mother got back on her feet just enough to work, she'd leave the aid behind. I imagine that had to do with the way everyone around her told her she was being lazy and taking advantage of the situation, something many people with invisible diseases still hear today. Everybody thinks it can't be that bad, you must be faking or just a drama queen. Yes, she was a drama queen, but she wasn't faking. Her illness was very real. Every time the work stress and hours became too much, she'd get sick again. We'd have to start the process from scratch—petitions, paperwork, waiting on approvals—all while watching her health decline. Meanwhile, the bills went unpaid until the benefits started again.

But that was what she wanted. It was her one small show of independence, her way of saying, "I'm not dead yet. I'm still contributing. I still matter." And I get it. She didn't want to give up all control. She didn't want to feel useless. After all, she was only in her 30s at this point, living with a disease that didn't even have a name when she was first diagnosed.

And health insurance? She only had it briefly when she worked at a law firm in New Orleans in the '90s. The minute they suspected she was sick and got wind that she was suing a local hospital, they let her go, which was perfectly (if not ethically) legal back then. So her entire life and my childhood were lived without insurance, backup plans, or a safety net. She had me and whatever patchwork support we could string together.

Why I Do What I Do

The contrast between how we approach chronic illness today versus the 1960s and 1970s is staggering. Today, we have disability insurance, long-term care coverage, critical illness riders, and wraparound products that can fill in the gaps when life falls apart. Health insurance is more readily available, and it's illegal to fire someone because of their health.

When I look back at my childhood and the challenges my mother and I faced because of her chronic illness, I can see the gaps and holes that could have been filled by insurance products that are available today. Back then, nobody sat down with you and explained your options. Nobody said, "Hey, if you had this policy in place, you wouldn't have to make life-and-death decisions based on what's in (or in our case, what's *not* in) your bank account."

People ask me all the time how I got into financial planning. I always tell them the truth: I lived through the consequences of not having a financial plan. My mother spent most of her life sick, uninsured, and one paycheck—or one lousy hospital visit—away from total disaster. And when she got sick? We had nothing. No coverage. No safety net. That's why I went into this business. Because if even *one* of the tools I help people secure today had been available—or more importantly, *used*—back then, my life and hers could've looked entirely different.

So now, I help people find their blind spots by asking the hard questions. I say, "What happens if you're in a wreck tomorrow and can't work for six months?" Or "If your spouse had a stroke, could you afford to keep them at home?" Most people don't think about those things. Or they think they'll handle it if it comes up. But trust me—when you need a plan, it's too late to make one.

I once had a lovely couple in their late 60s and 70s reach out to me. Their son was a reporter in New Orleans, and he had told them, "You need to talk to someone about long-term care." So they did. They called MetLife, and I happened to be the agent on duty.

I went to their house and sat at their kitchen table, ready to walk them through everything. But the husband was such a jokester. He was one of those guys with fake buttons on the wall and silly gadgets that squirted water at you when you weren't looking. He kept cracking jokes and couldn't take the conversation seriously. His wife, on the other hand, was dead serious. She wanted coverage. She knew what could happen, but I couldn't get through to him.

About a year later, my phone rang. It was him, and this time, he wasn't laughing.

"Shelly, can I still get that policy for my wife?"

"Well, can I talk to her?" I asked.

He paused, then said quietly, "No...she had a stroke. She's in a nursing home, and I can't afford to keep her there anymore."

My heart sank because by then, it was too late. The coverage he'd joked his way out of could've saved them financially. Instead, I helped him apply for Medicaid. He had to spend nearly all of their assets just to qualify. He was allowed to keep $80,000 total and keep his primary home, but he could never drive a car newer than 4 years old. That was it. I'll never forget the way he cried on the phone.

That's why I do what I do and say what I say. I'm pretty blunt and bold, which may sometimes make people uncomfortable. But sugarcoating what happens when life shows up uninvited and unplanned doesn't change what happens.

Think This Won't Happen to You?

If you're reading this and thinking, "That won't happen to me," I hope you're right. Many people think that way. But hope is not a strategy, and I'd rather be the person who made you uncomfortable by making you think about your potential future reality now than the one holding your hand when it's too late to change the outcome. I work with people of all ages, and I always say:

- If you love someone, you buy life insurance.

- If you love *yourself*, you buy disability insurance.
- If you care about your dignity, you make sure someone else doesn't have to wipe your ass someday because you failed to plan for long-term care.

After all of these years in financial planning, I can tell you exactly why people don't get the insurance coverage they need. There are only four reasons, and I've seen every one of them up close.

1. No time to talk about it.
2. No money to buy it.
3. No health to be able to obtain it .
4. No one they love that they'd want to preserve the dignity of (including themselves) during the worst of their physical and emotional health, nor are they responsible for providing for anyone beyond their death.

That's it. That's the whole list. And honestly, it's not necessarily that they don't have enough insurance. Often, people have too much of the wrong kind and not enough of what they need, and they just don't know what they don't know. That's where someone like me comes in.

I don't sell my clients coverage they don't need. But I do make sure they don't end up like my mom—fighting for their lives while worrying how they're going to pay for the next round of medication, the next home health aide, or the next month of care in a nursing home. I help people protect what they've built. I help them sleep at night. Because I know firsthand what it looks like when you're not protected correctly.

If you're not sure what kind of coverage you have, let me tell you something—you're not alone. Most people have no idea what they're paying for. And even less know whether it's the right kind of coverage for their current situation. It's not just about whether you have insurance. It's whether you have the right type, in the right amount, at the right time.

I've met people who are 55 years old, sitting on a $3 million life insurance policy—and no long-term care plan, disability coverage, or way to cover care if they have a stroke next week. When I ask them why they have so much life insurance, they usually say, "Well, I bought it years ago when the kids were little, and I never looked at it again."

Okay, but what about *now*? Are your kids still dependent on you? Are you carrying that same level of debt? Or are you about to become a burden to them because you don't have a plan for aging or illness?

The biggest mistake you can make is not knowing what you've got and finding out too late that it's not enough. And if you're relying on your employer coverage? Employer disability covers 60%, maybe 70% of your income, and it's taxable. So all in all, it only provides you with about 50% of your earnings.

If you don't know what you have, start by pulling out your policies. Dust them off and call your agent if you remember who they are. Sit down with someone who will explain it in plain English, not insurance jargon. And if you don't want to talk to anyone yet? Fine. At least start reading. Go to a reputable website and look up articles. Use the calculators. Educate yourself.

Need a starting point? Check out the website for this book, where you can access a whole library of resources. No pressure, no pitch. Just information. You don't have to get it perfect. You just have to get started. The only thing worse than planning for the worst is not preparing at all.

Being a caregiver isn't easy, and that's something I figured out from a very young age. Anything you can do today to help support yourself on this journey will be helpful. The day-to-day responsibilities of caregiving are heavy. In the next chapter, I'll give you an inside look at what it was like for me.

Chapter 3

What's a Normal Childhood?

L ooking back at my childhood today, I'm shocked at how
many everyday childhood experiences I never had.

There were no backyard barbecues with family, neighbors,
or friends. Cousins might have come in over the summer, or
gone out to my Aunt Lola and Uncle Marlin's house in Pleasant
Valley and eaten homemade ice cream, but those were extra
special days and never a guarantee.

High school dances? The only time I ever went to one was just
to walk through the breezeway to find someone I had been
looking for the night of the dance. My mom never dropped me
off at the mall, slipped me a twenty, and told me to "have fun."
If you could flip through my childhood like a photo album,
you'd find gaps where all those everyday "normal" moments
should be.

I didn't know my childhood was any different from any other
kid when I was little. When you're 5 or 6, you naturally assume
that whatever you're experiencing *is* normal because it's all
you know. But when I started going to school and spending
time around other kids, the differences began to show. Other
kids had parents who showed up at the school to drop off

forgotten permission slips, or sat in the bleachers for their games, or extracurricular school events. I didn't have that level of support. I wasn't even involved in extracurricular events, as my transportation wasn't dependable. I had a mom who was either too sick to leave the house or trying to gather enough strength just to get through the day.

At home, "normal" meant being told, "No, I can't take you, I'm not feeling well," or "I'm taking a nap" when I asked for a ride or help with something. My life revolved around her illness. If she were having a better day, maybe we'd play. If it were the day the clerk of court cut the child support check, we'd drive over to Canyon to pick it up. Sometimes she'd take me to a matinee movie afterwards.

While other kids my age were thinking about homework, boyfriends, and football games, I was thinking about whether or not Mom would be feeling well when she woke up in the morning…or whether she'd wake up at all. Every day had a question mark on it, and every answer depended on her health.

The Everyday Reality of a Sick Parent

My mom's illness wasn't the kind you could schedule things around. Crohn's doesn't have neat cycles or predictable flare-ups. It was a constant, uninvited houseguest that dictated everything from when we could go somewhere to who could come over and even what mood the day might take.

Back in the '70s, ileitis (Crohn's) disease wasn't something your average person—even doctors—knew about. In fact, in many places, it wasn't even called Crohn's until well into the '70s.

Today, there are specialists, treatment plans, and a whole host of medication options. But back then, it felt like there were only two options: You went into the hospital to die, or you went home and learned to live with it until you died...but she lived.

The "treatment" plan doctors recommended to my mom included telling her not to eat spicy, greasy, or fried food. Try that in West Texas! We invented Tex-Mex, chicken-fried steak, and calf fries. In 1956, that was over half of every menu in town! As for home cooking, I assure you there was nothing about farm-to-table that didn't include lard, sugar, flour, and cornmeal in my family's recipes. I'm not sure what she ate when she first got diagnosed—I was too young to think to ask.

Medical professionals provided these instructions to try to limit my mom's episodes of pain and discomfort. As it was, Dr. Dine was prescribing maximum amounts of prednisone. In the end, that would be more prednisone than she could maintain safely, and she was hoping the inflammation would calm down. Oh, and she was supposed to avoid stressful situations too!

Do you think any—and I do mean *any*—18-year-old girl who has just been told they have terminal ileitis knows how to handle the news? At that time, there had been no other reported cases of said condition in a female in the United States. Only four males in the Northeast had been diagnosed and received treatment. No one knew what to do about the disease or how to treat it. Could she honestly be expected to "avoid stressful situations"? I used to ask her what planet her doctors were from because there was no way they could be from the planet of Texas! She was only the fifth documented case diagnosed. Give me a break!

Nobody was talking about nutrition, remission, or long-term management. Most of the nurses and doctors we saw had never even heard of ileitis (Crohn's) disease before meeting my mom. The medical community only referred to it as ileitis until Dr. Crohn started authoring medical papers and dug in and began to research this dreadful disease. The doctors had to figure it out in real time right alongside us. It was a whole lot of guesswork, a little bit of luck, and a lot of just getting through the day.

Most mornings, I woke up wondering if she'd be alive. That sounds dramatic, but it was true. Even as a very young child, I never went to bed with the peace of mind that the next day would be simple. There was no guarantee of breakfast, no steady routine of school, home, and dinner. Every day was a roll of the dice, and I learned early that if I wanted some certainty in my life, I'd have to create it myself.

If Mom was too sick, there were no errands, no school drop-offs, no quick runs to the store. "No" was the answer more often than not. I heard these phrases all throughout my childhood:

"No, I can't take you."

"No, I'm not feeling well."

"No, I'm too tired."

Every "no" signified more than just a physical absence. Each "no" was a reminder that any plans I had could dissolve in an instant.

That kind of uncertainty changes you. I became hyperaware, constantly scanning for signs of how bad things might be that day. Was she in bed? In the bathroom? Was she pale or in pain? I learned to read her face and her voice like a meteorologist reads the weather forecast. When I could see the storm coming, I adjusted by canceling my plans, keeping quiet, and handling what needed handling.

Over time, every issue started to feel like life or death because for us, it often was. There was no "just a bad day." There were only good days, and then there were days when everything could fall apart.

Becoming the Caregiver

Some kids grow up playing house. I grew up running one.

When my mom didn't feel well—and that was most days—I stepped in without even realizing it was unusual. After each hospitalization, I fed her baby food in bed. Each hospitalization usually meant she'd had another resection of her small intestine and would be unable to digest adult food for a while. She would come home and have to eat baby food until her intestines had healed enough to tolerate more solid foods introduced over time.

The Gerber plums and apricots were our favorite flavors of baby food. I'd give her a spoonful, then take one for myself. One for her, one for me. It was the one thing about it that we both enjoyed. It was expensive to feed an adult enough baby food to survive on, so we really stretched it out.

I made her breakfast in bed too—but not because it was a special occasion. Once, when I'd spent the night at a friend's house, her mom served us breakfast in bed in the morning. I thought that was so nice that I went home and occasionally served breakfast to my mom in bed.

My mom spent hours at a time in the bathroom, lying on the floor with a heating pad on her stomach. When she was having a flare-up, she'd be on the toilet until there was nothing else to do. I'd often lie on the floor with her as she stayed in the bathroom all night.

I was the one who did the clean-up when she was too weak to make it to the bathroom in time. One of the reasons she didn't leave the house much was that she never knew when she was going to have a bowel movement or how far away the bathroom would be when she needed one. One of the most significant ways I took care of her was by not making her go anywhere.

When there weren't other kids living on the block—and there often weren't—my only playmate was my mom. I'd beg her to play with me. We'd watch movies together, play with my dolls, or just keep each other company. Sometimes caregiving wasn't about chores at all. Sometimes it was about being her best friend because she didn't have the strength to go out and be anyone else's. When times were good, she'd let me miss school for the day so we could play. Sometimes she would even take me out of school to go to the movies or to Nashville! Outside of that, she basically lived inside the house and didn't go anywhere or do anything when she was sick.

When she was well, the entire script flipped. She worked unconventional jobs. She was a weather girl and a copywriter at an ad agency. She also had a midnight radio show called

"Teena's Nightcap," where she read the short stories and poetry she authored.

Country singer Mel Tillis owned the radio station she worked for at that time. She couldn't pay a sitter, so she brought me with her and made me a pallet under the mixing board for me to sleep on until she got off.

During a good two-year run, she ran a production company that booked entertainment to come to Amarillo and perform in the Civic Center. I would get to be backstage with her, getting autographs. She brought Buck Owens and the entire Hee Haw gang (including Dolly Parton) to town. That was fun, but short-lived.

My mother also wrote music. When Buck was in Amarillo, she played several demos for him, one of which he seemed to like. He agreed to take the demo with him and let a couple of folks back in Nashville hear it. Mom was thrilled! About six months later, Mom and I were driving home after she picked me up from school. Suddenly, she slammed on the brakes and turned up the volume on the car radio. Coming through the car's speaker was Gladys Knight singing a beautiful song. After a moment or two, my mom started to sing with her, only occasionally missing a word here and there. When the song finished, she calmly stated, "That son of a bitch stole my record," referring to Buck Owens.

Mom would later find out that the attorney she hired to file the trademark paperwork for her publishing company had decided to stop off for a drink at his favorite local bar on the way back to the office and bought a round for the bar using the $100 she'd paid him. Because he never did his job, her subsequent method of copyrighting the demo (mailing a certified copy to herself) was invalid.

With all of these types of things happening all the time in my daily life as a child, my philosophy as an adult has been (after starting therapy, mind you), "Calm down. Is anybody gonna die from this? If they're not, then we can work out all of this. I'm not saying it won't be painful, or terrible, and/or hard, but if no one's going to die, we're golden." No issue was "only" terrible or critical for us when I was a kid, though. Life always hung in the balance, every single day—not just hers, but mine too.

So I learned to be adaptable, but not because I was easygoing (I'm not). I saw early on that every day could change without warning. Making plans was a luxury I didn't have. I had to be flexible just to survive. I also learned that if I needed something, I had to be able to provide it for myself.

Providing for Myself

I was always in charge of myself. There was never a day when someone else was going to swoop in and make sure my lunch money was in my pocket or my laundry was folded and put away. I learned how to do the laundry at age 6 so that if I needed clean clothes, I could make it happen. If I needed lunch money and there wasn't any in the house, I went hunting for Coke bottles to turn in for a nickel apiece at the Toot'n Totem five blocks away.

Sometimes my mom would call my dad and ask him to bring over some lunch money—or at least Coke bottles from the machine at his office—but that usually turned into an argument. He'd ask her what frivolous thing she had spent the child support on this time, which was laughable because he only paid $150 a month at the time. She was either working sporadically, temporarily, or not at all, depending on the level of flare-up she was having. Many times, that $150 was all we had to live on.

I learned how to work the washer and dryer young—so young that one time, I decided to "dry" the cat after I accidentally got it wet in the backyard at my grandmother's house. I shut the cat in the dryer, turned it on, and stood there until my grandmother came running when she heard the thumping and loud meows. I told her exactly what happened. She sighed, then told me to stand back. When she opened the door, the cat shot out of that dryer like a rocket. She calmly informed me that cats can't go in dryers because they'll shrink, and I believed her.

That wasn't my only early experiment in bad decision-making. Around age 3, during naptime, I decided it was the perfect time to try smoking. I knew I wasn't supposed to, so I snuck into the living room with a match and a cigarette, hid behind the big chair, and lit up. The match burned my finger, and I dropped it. Unbeknownst to me, the carpet and drapes caught fire as I ran to tell my mother I needed a bandage. The fire department had to come, and my secret was out.

I walked everywhere until I was 10, when we finally scraped together enough money for a kelly green 10-speed Schwinn from Hill's Bike Shop. I hated that color, but it was what we could afford, and the owner let my mom pay for it over time. It cost $131—a fortune in 1974—and I rode it until I left home.

By the time I was 9, I'd started babysitting, and my earnings went straight to my mom for groceries. By age 13, I had regular jobs, which my friend Cindy down the street sometimes referred me to. But even then, my ability to work depended on whether Mom felt well enough to drive me there. If she couldn't, I stayed home. My ability to earn, to go anywhere, even to be a kid, was always tied to her health.

It didn't feel strange at the time. It was just the way life worked—if I wanted or needed something, I found a way to handle it myself.

Emotional and Social Costs

The hardest part wasn't the chores or the Coke bottle hunts. It was the way my mom's illness kept me on the sidelines of what other kids my age were doing. I missed a lot of school. I was late more than I was on time. I showed up without permission slips, missed announcements, and sometimes didn't even know about school events until they'd already happened.

That kind of inconsistency has a way of closing doors before you even know they're there. I didn't go to a single high school dance. Not one. Opportunities passed me by because I wasn't present enough—or reliable enough in the eyes of the adults making decisions. Even though I was relatively popular, well-liked, and good at something, there was always the unspoken question: Can she show up for this?

One of the clearest examples of that came when I tried out for the junior high cheerleading squad (everything middle school was referred to as junior high in the 70s in Texas). I'll save the whole story for chapter 6, but let's just say my absences and my mom's illness played a significant role in how that turned out. And it hurt—not just because I didn't make it, but because I realized my life at home had the power to shape my world outside of it.

Those years taught me to expect disappointment, to assume things might not work out, and to be ready to roll with it when they didn't. It was a survival skill, but it came at the cost of a lot of the "normal" teenage experiences other kids took for granted.

Growing Up Surrounded by Caregivers

Looking back, it's no surprise I slipped so naturally into a caregiving role. I come from a long line of women who did the same. Both of my grandmothers were nurses. My grandmother on my dad's side graduated in the very first nursing class at St. Anthony's Hospital—one of only six women in the program— and she worked almost until the day she died of breast cancer at just 52. My grandmother on my mom's side didn't become a nurse until she was 39 or 40, well after my mom was diagnosed with Crohn's. She went on to be the charge nurse at the local nursing home, the same place my great-grandmother lived out her last years.

The thing is, my caregiving at home didn't look like what they did in the hospital. I wasn't changing IVs or taking blood pressure, at least not yet. My "nursing" was doing endless loads of laundry, keeping my mom company, or even cleaning up an accident on the bathroom floor while she lay there with a heating pad, waiting for the pain to pass. Sometimes it was as simple—and as heavy—as making sure she didn't feel alone when she was too sick to move.

It wasn't medical training, but it was caregiving all the same. And even though I didn't think of it that way at the time, those years shaped how I saw myself: capable, responsible, and always ready to step in when someone else couldn't keep going.

And my mother was sacrificing just as much as I was. With all my heart and soul, I fully believe that the reason she stayed alive so long was to take care of me. I know there were times she was tired and in pain and just didn't want to do it anymore. Then this happy little girl (me) would come bouncing into the room.

"Hey, Mom! What can I do for you? What can I get you? How can I help?"

She didn't want to leave that happy little girl alone.

Lessons in Resilience

By the time most kids my age were just figuring out how to drive, I already knew how to run a household, manage a crisis, and make decisions no 13-year-old should have to make. My worth—at least how I understood it—was tied to keeping my mom alive and as comfortable as possible. People told me what a wonderful caregiver I was, and I believed them. That praise became part of who I was.

The problem is, when you learn early that your value comes from meeting other people's needs, it's hard to turn that off. Even later, when I had children of my own—one with special needs and one without—I carried that same relentless drive to make sure neither of them "missed a beat," no matter what it cost me. I worked myself to the bone, went 15 years without remarrying, and rarely asked for help because the school of hard knocks had informally trained me to expect to handle it all on my own.

Those years with my mom gave me skills that served me well—adaptability, resourcefulness, and the ability to keep calm in the middle of chaos. But those years also made it hard to trust others to show up for me. I didn't even know what help to ask for. I'd seen nothing to the contrary, so I came to believe help wasn't coming. Disappointment had been the norm for so long that it felt safer to just plan around it.

Resilience is a good thing—until you realize it's costing you the chance to be cared for too.

Doing Things Differently

If there's one thing I know now that I wish everyone back then had understood, it's that we all could have done better—myself included. My mom's illness was a first for everyone in our world. Most of the doctors and nurses we saw had never treated Crohn's before, and outside the big cities, many still called it just ileitis. Treatment was more guesswork than science, and the best advice she usually got was, "Don't eat and rest." Nobody was talking about long-term nutrition, emotional support, or what it meant for a child to grow up as a caregiver.

That's why I believe so strongly in meeting people where they are now. It's not about blame—it's about awareness. Teachers, neighbors, friends, coaches…somebody has to notice when a kid is carrying more than their share and step in with the right kind of help. Sometimes that means bending the rules. Sometimes it just means listening.

Every day, you see posts shared on social media regarding how autoimmune diseases are still looked at as silent diseases. A person seems perfectly normal, so that must mean they are just lazy, or dramatic, or a liar. My mother was none of those things, but try to tell someone that when the patient they're looking at is literally *the first female.*

So no, my childhood wasn't easy. And I didn't know it then, but life was about to hand me a whole new challenge—one that had nothing to do with my mom's illness. If I thought I'd learned how to adapt, the arrival of my stepmonster was about to put that to the test.

Chapter 4

The Evil Stepmonster

F ive or six months after my parents decided not to remarry a third time, my father met the woman I'll call Stepmonster.

At first, this woman seemed fine. She even gave me a school bus lunchbox before my first day of second grade. I adored that lunchbox, and I felt so special and loved. Unfortunately, it was all an act. Once she had my father, she didn't need to pretend anymore. She made it quickly apparent that I wasn't welcome. I wasn't part of the family. I was just an inconvenient guest. And just like that, my father's house—the only place that had ever felt *almost* safe—was ruined.

Parents Without Partners

My father was a lot of things—disciplined, structured, practical—but one thing he was *not* was someone who liked being alone. For a man who had spent most of his life in environments that demanded self-sufficiency—boarding school, the Navy, Texas A&M, running his own business— you'd think he would have been fine on his own. But he wasn't.

Maybe it was because he never really *had* to be alone. He went from his parents' house to military school, to the Navy, to a dorm at A&M. The only time in his life when he didn't have someone built into his daily routine was after each divorce. And he must have decided he didn't like it much because after that, he was always looking for someone to fill the space beside him.

He started going to these events for a group called Parents Without Partners. It was exactly what it sounded like—a club for single parents who didn't want to be single anymore. I guess it was the 1970s version of online dating, except instead of swiping right, you had to show up to places and talk to people in real life.

He dated, of course. A lot. Some of them I met, some of them I didn't. But there's one woman I *do* remember—Mrs. Maxwell. I don't remember her first name. None of my other relatives, including my uncle and my brother, even remember her. But I do. I remember her because I *liked* her.

It's strange when you're a kid watching your parents date. It's even stranger when you're a kid who has already faced significant challenges and heartbreak. But Mrs. Maxwell was different.

The first time I met her, my dad picked me up on a Saturday morning and said, "Do you mind stopping by Mrs. Maxwell's house for coffee?" I was always up for anything on those rat-killing mornings—I didn't cause trouble or throw fits—so I just nodded and went along with it.

We arrived, and she welcomed us like she'd been expecting us. She made coffee for my dad from the container of Maxwell House on the counter, and I sat at her kitchen table, watching them talk. She was warm. Kind. The sort of woman who made you feel like you belonged just by how she looked at you.

And because I was almost 6 and didn't have much of a filter, I asked the first question that popped into my head, "Is Maxwell House *your* coffee?"

She laughed. My dad laughed. And even though the answer was no, she didn't make me feel stupid for asking. She smiled and said, "I wish it were, sweetheart."

I don't know what happened between her and my dad, but I never saw her again for whatever reason. My dad kept dating. And then one day, he came home with *her*—my stepmonster.

I wondered what my life would have been like if Daddy had married Mrs. Maxwell instead. It would have been different. Better. But that wasn't what happened. Instead, he kept looking. He kept showing up at Parents Without Partners activities and events, trying to find someone who would fit into his life as he needed them to. And that's how I ended up in Colorado Springs at some kind of organized camp getaway for single parents and their kids to mix, mingle, and see if they could form new little families. I don't remember much about that weekend, but I do know that's where I met my stepmonster for the first time.

She was just another face in the crowd then—one of the many women who fluttered around my father, laughing too loudly at his jokes and making polite conversation. My father was successful and established, but he was not a handsome man. So when women flocked to him, that made him uncomfortable.

I think, deep down, he always worried that women weren't actually interested in *him*—just what he could provide.

There used to be this cologne back in the '70s called High Karate. The commercials made it seem as if a man put it on, women would lose their damn minds. They'd chase him through the streets, unable to control themselves. Well, someone—one of the women there, I assume—had bought my dad a bottle of it. And for some reason, he decided this would be the perfect time to put some on.

We were all in the camp's fellowship hall, a big open space where people were eating, talking, and flirting. When the women noticed he was wearing High Karate, they re-enacted the commercial.

They started chasing him.

Not just playfully, either. They were *really* chasing him like he was the last eligible man on Earth.

My daddy panicked. He bolted straight for the bathroom, ran inside, and locked the door behind him. Not discouraged, the women started banging on the door, telling him to come out.

He refused, and that's when they sent me in.

One of the women turned to me and said, "Go knock on the door and tell him to come out."

I felt special that they'd asked me, so I did. I knocked and called out, "Daddy?"

The door cracked open just enough for him to grab me by the arm and pull me inside before slamming it shut again. We stood in that tiny bathroom, just the two of us, the sounds of giggling women outside.

And I remember looking up at him and saying, "Well, we can't let you wear that cologne anymore."

He just shook his head, exasperated. That was my dad. He wanted the attention. They appeared to be attracted to him, but he was never sure why. I just never felt like he was ever comfortable or entirely at ease with it. He was always searching for something he wasn't even sure how to define. Ultimately, he picked the wrong woman, and my life was never the same.

Becoming Excess Baggage

When she first came into my life, Stepmonster was all smiles and fake kindness, the kind of woman who knew exactly how to play the part—at least when people were watching. Stepmonster had a soft voice, a polished look, and an air that made people assume she was charming and refined. She was a woman who knew how to host a dinner party and balance a checkbook without a hair out of place.

And in those first few months, she played her role well. Remember how I said she gave me a brand-new lunchbox before my first day of second grade? At the time, I thought, *She likes me! She thinks I'm special!*

But that thought didn't last long. Once she had my father, once the marriage certificate and prenup were signed, and the wedding was over, the act was over too. She didn't need to be nice to me anymore. She'd gotten what she wanted—the man, the house, the position of Mrs. Grimm. And I was just…excess baggage. A leftover piece of his past life that she had to tolerate. From then on, every interaction with her made it clear—I was an inconvenience.

I still remember the day I realized, beyond a shadow of a doubt, that I couldn't count on her.

I was 7 years old. By then, my mother had recovered enough to start working temp jobs again while I was at school. One school day, something must have happened at the temp job to hold her up because for whatever reason, she couldn't pick me up after school. She called the office and told them to call my dad. In those days, there wasn't anything like after-school care. Shoot, most moms weren't even working yet unless they were the primary breadwinner, single, or their husband's income didn't take care of all the household needs. What I'm trying to say is, it wasn't uncommon AT ALL for women to stay home and be homemakers. Anyway, Daddy sometimes picked me up at school since my mom was sick so much. I sat in the front office, waiting while they dialed. His secretary answered.

"He's in a meeting," she said. "I don't know when he'll be available."

The school secretary and I decided to wait a little while, and then we'd try to call back. After about 15 minutes, we tried to reach my dad again and were told that he wouldn't be out of his meeting for another hour or so.

Okay. That was fine. Stepmonster was next on the contact list. I didn't particularly *want* a ride home with her, but she had a pretty cushy job and had been able to get off to pick me up before. At least she'd come and get me, right? Wrong.

I sat there, listening as school secretary made the call.

"Hi, this is the secretary from Michelle's school. I'm calling because you are one of the contacts listed to come pick her up. We received a message that her mother is at work and her father is in a meeting. She needs someone to come pick her up. What would you like me to do with her?"

"Well, she'll just have to wait until one of them can come get her. Let me talk to her," Stepmonster demanded, her clipped, annoyed voice audible through the phone.

The school secretary frowned and then handed me the phone.

"I'm at work," Stepmonster said. "I can't come get you. You're going to have to make other arrangements now."

Dejected, I handed the phone back to the secretary. Then I heard Stepmonster make one final request.

"Take me off the contact list."

And just like that, she was off the phone. No hesitation. No "Oh, I wish I could, but I just can't get away" or "Let me see if I can get through to your father." Just no.

I sat there for what felt like forever. The school emptied as kids were picked up one by one. The teachers and principal left, and the secretaries started packing their things.

At some point, I realized no one was coming for me, and I wasn't waiting anymore, so I did the only thing I *could*: I started walking.

The Long Walk Home

The school wasn't terribly from my house—just three miles—but that was a decent distance for a 7-year-old. I did it though. I carried that stupid school bus lunchbox and walked home alone down one of the busiest streets in town.

I made stops along the way. First, I stopped at a schoolmate's house—I swear this girl was the original mean girl. I hoped her mother, who was the Brownie leader, would let me use the phone, but I didn't even get a chance to ask because the mean girl said no and slammed the door in my face.

I saw a church across the street that I'd been to a few times. Maybe I could use their phone. But nobody was there, so I kept walking.

The thing is, I didn't even cry. I wasn't scared. I wasn't panicking. Deep down, I think I already knew something was wrong, and this situation confirmed what I had suspected for a long time: I was on *my own*.

I walked those three miles like it was just another part of my day, my little legs carrying me through neighborhoods and across intersections, past stores and houses where other kids were probably sitting at the dinner table, eating food someone had cooked for them. I must have been quite a sight—a tiny 7-year-old walking down a major road with a lunchbox—but no one stopped to see if I was okay.

When I finally made it home, nobody was there. Nobody had been looking for me. When my mother eventually got home, she never asked how I got home. She just assumed my father had picked me up. And my father? He never asked either.

Nobody even knew that I had walked home alone. That was the moment I understood exactly where I stood in the world.

It wasn't only that my stepmonster didn't care about me—it was that nobody was going to fight for me. Not my mother, who was too caught up in her own struggles. Not my father, who always chose whatever was easiest. Not the teachers at my school, who assumed someone would eventually show up. I was an afterthought. I had no safety net. No fallback. No home base where I could land if things got bad.

My stepmonster had made sure of that. She hadn't just refused to pick me up; she had gone out of her way to ensure she was never responsible for me again. She had erased herself from my life in the most intentional way possible.

From that moment on, I knew—I couldn't count on anyone but myself.

The Takeover

It wasn't enough for Stepmonster to clarify that I was not welcome.

She wanted me gone, and not just me. My brother lived with my dad when she moved in, and no love was lost between them. She saw him as nothing but a problem, a disruption, a stain on the picture-perfect life she had planned for herself. He was often gone and shipped out to some program, school, or another. But she started pushing, needling, and creating fights when he was home. One day, she got exactly what she wanted—he hit her.

I don't condone violence, but I also know my brother. I know how much she provoked him, how she got in his face, poked and prodded, and told him flat out, "I've already managed to get visitation with your sister down to only a day or two. Now I'm going to get you out."

That's when he snapped. One punch was all it took. My father came home that night, walked downstairs to where my brother was already packing his things, and said, "Well, I guess you know what has to happen now, huh?"

He knew. He was just waiting for Dad to say he was out.

That was it. He spent the second half of his senior year of high school living out of his car. Remember now, that's January through May. Those can be some pretty brutal nights in January through March. He couch surfed when he could and made do in the freezing cold when he couldn't.

Stepmonster was thrilled—one down, one to go.

Once my brother was out of the house, she thought I'd be easier to eliminate. I was smaller and younger. How much of a threat could I be? But she underestimated me. I had been fighting for my place since I was old enough to understand loneliness. I knew how to exist in the shadows and make myself small enough to stay under the radar. I learned how to survive.

After all, I'd been collecting cans and turning them in for lunch money for years—I grew up before the days of free school lunches. But that didn't mean I had a safe place to call home.

My mother loved me, but she was a horrible parent, and sometimes she was too sick to take care of me. My grandmother had never been the nurturing type. And my father had chosen his new wife over me without a second thought.

The part of my father that had been mine was taken away by my stepmonster, and she had several ways of making sure I knew it. Like the way she always insisted on answering the phone first and making me ask if I could talk to my dad.

It wasn't enough for her to have my father. It wasn't enough that she had pushed my brother out of the house, made their home an unwelcoming place, and ensured that my father's attention belonged solely to her. No, she needed more. She needed control, which meant making sure I—a kid who never asked for any of this—knew exactly where I stood.

Even worse, my dad went along with it. I'll never forget the day we were on our way to his house on a Saturday afternoon, and he said, "Your stepmother is feeling like you don't like her."

Who? Me? I was a kid who had more than most adults did on my plate.

"When we get to the house, before you go over to the little girls' house across the street to play, could you go in and talk to her?" he asked. "She just wants to feel included."

And because I was a good kid, because I still thought that maybe if I played by the rules, things would get better, I did what he asked. I walked into the living room, where she was already waiting for me, and sat next to her, listening as she told me how she wanted us to have a better relationship. She wanted me to feel like I could come to her. And then, she said the thing I knew was coming.

"You know, Michelle...you can call me Mom."

I felt my whole body go stiff. My mother may have been sick. She may not have been the most incredible parent or the easiest person to live with. But she was still my mother. I looked her dead in the eye with all the butter-wouldn't-melt-in-my-mouth coolness and enough sweetness to evoke a diabetic coma and shared the one thing I had to say to that: "That won't be necessary. I have one, thank you."

From that moment on, there was no possibility of a happy little stepmonster-stepdaughter relationship. She knew it, and I knew it. When I went to their house, I had to knock on the front door as a guest and greet her first before I could see my dad or play with the little girls who lived across the street. I had to formally acknowledge her presence as if she were some kind of queen perched on her throne.

After the stepmonster came into the picture—even when my brother was away—my dad's house was no longer an option. It wasn't a place I could go to escape, to reset, or to feel safe. When I needed that kind of help, he couldn't give it to me. She made sure of it. The moment Stepmonster walked into my father's life, my fate was sealed. There would be no safety net for me. No welcome mat was waiting at the door.

Doing Things Differently

It's easy to sit here years later and wonder how things could have gone differently. If one choice or one decision had been made another way, would my life have turned out the same? Would I have still been the kid walking home alone from school? The child who had no place where she was allowed to be a kid? Would I have still learned how to fend for myself before I knew what that meant? Or could things have been different?

I've concluded that if things had been different for me, I would have needed different people in my life.

If my father had stood up to Stepmonster and refused to allow her to control his relationships with his kids, maybe he would have been able to love me in ways that didn't require me to perform a ritual of acknowledging his wife before I could speak to him. Maybe I would have had a safe place to land. The result was the same, whether it was because he was afraid of being alone or because he convinced himself it was easier just to keep the peace. He chose her, at least during my childhood. Much later, he stood up for me and tried to make things right, but that's another story for another book.

If my mother hadn't needed to be in control of everything—if she had let people help her instead of demanding that help be given only on her impossible terms—maybe I could have had a childhood instead of spending mine taking care of her. But my mother was Teena, the Duchess. She was the woman who demanded the world move at her pace, on her terms, and who would rather suffer than admit she needed help. I had to make the adjustment. I had to be the one to make sure she was okay, even when I *wasn't*.

There's no point in pretending that my stepmonster could be anyone other than who she was—the woman who went out of her way to push me out of my daddy's life. A different woman wouldn't have told my brother, "I got your sister's visitation down to a few days. Now I will work on getting rid of you too." A different woman wouldn't have erased herself from my school's contact list, so she'd never be responsible for me again. A different woman might not have loved me, but she wouldn't have actively made my life hell either. But at the end of the day, she was who she was.

I think about it sometimes. What if my dad had fought for me? What if he hadn't married Stepmonster? What if my mother had accepted more help? What if my grandmother had been more available to me and not just my sister?

How could things have been different?

I'm not sure. Years later, I had conversations with my grandmother, mother, and sister about what could have been done differently, but what's done is done. I made it. The experiences I had made me the person I am today. It prepared me for the mission I have to help others prepare for the caregiver life they may be experiencing. Throughout my career, I have helped so many families, business owners, and individuals with their protection needs, including long-term care insurance, in an effort to ensure that other kids don't have to experience what I did. It prepared me to tell my story in hopes that others will recognize ways to be the person a child in a caregiving role needs.

The journey taught me a lot about resilience and responsibility, but it also taught me about what was missing. I know how different things might have been if we'd had more support, community, and connection. That's why I want to talk about something I wish someone had told me back then.

If You Don't Have "Your People," Find Them

If there's one thing I want you to hear me say loud and clear, it's this: You're not meant to do life alone, *especially* if you're a caregiver. Back when I was growing up, support systems didn't exist outside of a person's bloodline. You had your people, and if your people didn't step up…you were just out of luck. People judged you if your family didn't take care of you. They certainly judged my mother. But we don't live in that world anymore.

We live in a world where families are scattered across the country, where people grow up and move away for work, school, or just to start over. We're more mobile and disconnected, forcing us to build community purposefully. If you don't have a strong support system, it's time to create one.

Start local. Check out your local Boys & Girls Club of America. See what's available through your local community centers or churches. If your child has a hobby—sports, music, even gaming—there's probably a group out there already formed and ready to welcome you.

Don't overlook support groups. There is a group for almost everything—chronic illness, caregiving, single parenting, financial recovery, and grief. You name it. Some are faith-based. Some are not. Some meet in person. Others are online.

But they do exist. I've even worked with organizations that support women who've been financially abused—because, yes, that's a thing. And yes, it's way more common than anyone talks about. That kind of isolation and manipulation is real. It's not their fault; they don't have to stay stuck.

A friend of mine is a special education teacher. She realized most of her students—kids with significant disabilities—never got to go on vacation. Their families just couldn't manage it. So what did she do? She started a camp. Every year, she raises the money herself and brings in other teachers and support staff. And every year, ten kids experience something they'd never have otherwise. That's the kind of go-getter you should be looking for.

That's what I mean when I say support is out there. But you do have to ask for it—look and risk putting yourself out there. Yes, there are scammers. Yes, some people will take advantage if they can. But some good people have been where you are and are dedicated to helping others come out the other side.

So, if you're feeling alone, unsupported, or stretched beyond your limit, please hear me: You are not meant to carry this all by yourself. Find your people. If you're unsure where to start, start with our website and contact us. We'll be happy to recommend some organizations in your area.

Chapter 5

Building Confidence for Life

I guess you could say I had a big personality, even as a little girl. I couldn't help but let my creativity out through storytelling. I loved the way a story could hold a room full of people captive. I loved how words could make people feel something, whether it was curiosity, laughter, or surprise. My stories could really fill a space and command attention. I knew how to perform before I could even spell the word. I thank God for that because I would need every ounce of that big personality in the years ahead.

My brother recalled this one instance when he was halfway through telling my daddy about a dance at school he'd gone to the night before—who was there, who he danced with, what everybody wore—when I couldn't help but jump in.

"Well, I went to a dance last night too, Daddy," 4-year-old me interrupted.

I'd been listening to their exchange while we were riding in the car, sitting right in the middle of them in the front seat. We were heading out on one of those infamous Saturday morning "rat killing" adventures. Daddy had been nodding along and asking my brother questions. When I jumped in, he shifted his attention to me with a raised eyebrow and a big grin.

"Oh, you did? And who'd you dance with, Shotgun?" That was what my dad called me—Shotgun.

I spun up a big and sparkly description of my imagined event, complete with names, descriptions of beautiful dresses worn, punch flavors, the whole shebang. He let me finish, then, still smiling, leaned back in his seat and asked, "Now is any of that true?"

I shrugged and smiled. "Nope." I wasn't lying. I just love to tell a good story.

There were hard days coming—the kind that tried to shrink me down to nothing. Between my mother's illness and the stepmonster's overshadowing presence during the times I spent at my daddy's house, the light in me would flicker, threatening to go out more than once. Thankfully, I had someone in my corner who wasn't about to let me go into that fight unarmed—my mother.

My mother didn't have a maternal bone in her body. She told me later that she thought she could just give birth to my sister and me, and the rest would kind of take care of itself. Although Mom and I probably had the closest relationship out of anybody in my whole family—and I'm talking immediate *and* extended family—with her, there still weren't a lot of public displays of affection.

No one on my mother's side of the family exchanged hugs or kisses for except me. My grandmother was the matriarch who always insisted on being called "Grandmother." Not granny or grandma—any other derivative was utterly unacceptable. My grandmother was also a nurse who hated germs, so she wouldn't let anyone kiss her on the mouth either. Instead, she'd pop her cheek out with air and let you kiss her cheek.

Well, this loving, happy little girl wasn't having any of that! I would go in the house, pop her cheek with my finger, give her a quick peck on the lips, and say "Hi Granny!" She absolutely went bonkers…but on the inside, she absolutely loved it. That was our special deal.

When my grandmother died, I was the only one standing at that casket whom she had told more than twice that she loved them. I *made* her tell me. We had a routine when it was time to hang up on a phone call. I always started it.

"I love you, Grandmother," I'd say.

She'd respond, "I know you do."

"No, that's not the appropriate response to that statement," I'd say. "You're supposed to say, 'I love you too.'"

Then she would say something like "Well, I do."

That wasn't good enough for me. I'd pester her until she said it, then we'd hang up. After ten or so times, she fell into line, and saying "I love you" to each other became normal.

I didn't understand the significance of those interactions until the morning of my grandmother's funeral. I found my mother and sister crying in the TV room. I asked them why they were crying and hugging, which was very strange for them. They told me they were commiserating over how little they'd heard

"I love you" from Grandmother. My mom had heard it twice, and my sister once.

It was then that I stated very matter-of-factly: "Well, you don't have anybody to blame but yourself. I *made* her tell me she loved me every time I hung up the phone, ever since I moved away."

They were both floored. The grandchild who was disregarded—the one that got no support or individual time with my grandmother—how could it be that I was the one who had been told "I love you" by this stoic, responsible, hard-working, dependable woman regularly for the last two years? Because every time I talked to her, up to and including the day before she died, I had made it a part of our conversation. The two women I'm sure she loved most didn't get that honor because they didn't go first.

That's how I learned that if you want some kind of action or response from someone—be it emotional or physical—and they aren't providing it, you'd better speak up or your needs may not be met.

I cannot say that we should've expected great things from my mother's parenting skills, given her parents' lack of skill. And, although she may not have been the best parent, Mom did make sure I had confidence deep down in my bones. My mom saw not only who I was but also what I'd be up against. She wasn't sure how long she would be around, so she laid a foundation for my strong personality early.

When I was 7 or 8, my mother cut a record with a few songs. Her best friend for many years, Dee, sang on it. She had a lovely voice. I still have that record because my mother wrote one of the songs, "Summer Sunshine," for me.

The song they were promoting was called "Hereford Hustling Boomer Jump." It was a cute little ditty sung by another friend and business partner, Ray, with whom she had a production company called TeenaRay Productions, Inc. They booked music talent in town as another way to make money.

Through that production company, Mom had worked with most radio folks at some point, and those people all seemed to stick together. She'd already dropped records off at all the radio stations, but there were still about 100 records left. One day, she grabbed the box of records that was just gathering dust and said, "Come on, kid, we're going to Hereford to sell these."

After driving the 40 miles from Amarillo to Hereford, we pulled into a very nice residential neighborhood and found a place to park at the end of the block. She put me on one side of the street and before she took to the other side, she handed me five records.

"Go knock on those doors and see what you can do. Ask for $1."

It was just a little thing, but I did it. I walked right up to strangers' front doors, records in hand. And wouldn't you know it, I sold the only record that day. My mother always said I could sell ice to people in the Artic—and that afternoon, I proved her right.

Born for the Stage

My mother entered me in my first pageant when I was just 5 years old. When we lived in Oklahoma City, she worked for McCann Advertising, the sponsor of the "Our Little Miss Oklahoma" pageant. Although we had moved back to Amarillo by the time the pageant rolled around, Mom had recovered enough from her hospital stay to drive, so we went back to Oklahoma City for the pageant. At the time, I wasn't thinking about confidence or personal growth—I was thinking about the shiny crown and the sparkly dress. But not my mother. She was playing a much longer game.

She didn't care one bit if I won or lost. What she cared about was how comfortable I was on the stage. She wanted me to practice walking and looking people in the eyes as I did so. She cared that I felt comfortable when I walked across the stage. She wanted me to learn to command my presence in a way that let me own a room, whether in a church basement with balloons and crepe paper streamers or a civic center stage with spotlights and microphones.

I loved the stage, and Lord, the stage loved me. The more time I spent under the bright lights, the more I loved it, and my mother could tell. When she saw that I had a little sparkle in me, she didn't just let it flicker. She threw gasoline on it. She saw a big, bold personality in her little girl and thought, "What can I do to continue encouraging these qualities and traits in her? We'd better get that girl up on stage!"

Mother wrote ad copy, jingles, scripts, and screenplays for commercials and ad agencies in between Crohn's flare-ups.

Just like me, she knew how to get people to pay attention. She always had my sister and me star in the commercials she wrote—the ones that called for girls our age, anyway—and she encouraged me to get involved in school and community theater.

Looking back, I realize those pageants, commercials, and plays were training grounds. They helped me sharpen the skills I'd need to survive the emotional minefield that was my home life. I had a stepmonster who did everything she could to destroy my confidence, and a daddy who didn't know how to stand up for me without destroying his marriage. Mother knew what I dealt with at Daddy's. She didn't know how long she'd be with me. Putting me on the stage was one of her ways of putting steel in my spine. And when it came to her helping me build my confidence, she was just getting started.

Dr. Maxwell Maltz and the Mirror

The Christmas I was 8 years old, my mom gave me one of the most incredible gifts I have ever received—*Dr. Maxwell Maltz's Confidence Building Kit*. Of course, I didn't realize the impact it would have on me at the time. I thought it was really neat until I realized that was all I was going to get for Christmas. I'll let you guess how thrilled I was when I unwrapped my present, and there was this cardboard case and a bunch of cassette tapes. My mom tried to explain how, after I listened to these tapes and talked into the mirror centered neatly on the inside cover of the box, the "system" promised to build my self-esteem. As she spoke, I looked around under the tree, thinking that couldn't be all there was for me. It was. *What happened to the toys that had been on my Christmas list?* Other kids were unwrapping dolls and bikes, and I was building my self-esteem.

"That's it? That's my gift?" I asked. I didn't know who Dr. Maxwell Maltz was, but one thing I *did* know was who he *wasn't*—Santa Claus. Although his book, *Psycho-Cybernetics*, had been out for at least a decade by then, I was 8. I didn't know a thing about it, and I didn't have a clue about psycho-cybernetics.

"You still have Santa coming tonight," Mom replied. That gave me some hope. Surely he had all the goods. I'd just have to wait until morning.

When I woke up at my grandmother's house the following day, I ran into the living room to look under the tree. What I found confirmed right then was that there was no Santa Claus. I had the matching cassette tape recorder for that confidence-building kit—nothing more.

Those cassette tapes didn't just sit in the closet collecting dust. Mother made sure I put that cassette player to good use. I went through Dr. Maxwell Maltz's Confidence Building Kit cassette tape by cassette tape. Every day, I was supposed to pop in a tape and listen to Dr. Maltz's affirmations, like "You are confident. You are beautiful. You are worthy," and then stand in front of the mirror and repeat them.

I didn't understand it then, but looking back, I see what Mom was doing. She could have given me something fun that I would have played with for a time and then outgrown. Instead, she gave me something that helped build a strong foundation for my self-esteem. She knew that with everything going on in our lives—the chronic illness she battled, the back-and-forth hospital stays, the drama that came from my stepmonster—I was going to need to be strong just to survive. That kit became part of my routine the following year, like brushing my teeth or packing my school bag. Thank goodness I saw it as fun instead of a chore.

Over time, those affirmations started to sink in. Most moms back then taught their daughters to bake cookies or curl their hair. Mine was teaching me how to build neural pathways for resilience. That confidence-building kit taught me to stand firm and get back up when knocked down. I may have been disappointed and rolled my eyes about it as an 8-year-old, but today, I see how important it was. That confidence kit was more than a self-help tool—it was armor. And I discovered how to wear it well.

Learning the Games People Play

The summer I turned 12 was the summer everything shifted. Mom had deep connections in the Nashville-to-Hollywood scene. I remember sleeping on recording studio floors in Nashville while she and her best friend, Dee, cut records with people whose names you'd recognize. Through these connections, my mother was offered a chance to help finish a screenplay in California—*The Getaway*, with Steve McQueen and Ali MacGraw. It was a huge opportunity, and she couldn't pass it up. So she packed her bags and told me she'd get settled first. Then she would send for me at my grandmother's.

And she did. She stayed with her best friend, Delo, in La Jolla until she found an apartment of her own, and then she had me come to her. We did a lot in the first six days I was in California. We saw more in those six days than most folks do in six months. We visited the San Diego Zoo and took a quick hop to Tijuana. But then, reality set in.

Mom hadn't expected California to be quite so fast-paced, and it didn't seem to matter what neighborhood you lived in. This was back in the early '70s, during the height of the drug culture out there. You'd walk into a party and see bowls of coke on the coffee table in the living room. People walked around wearing coke spoons on strings or chains around their necks.

The last straw for her turned out to be when we were coming back from the zoo, and she saw this nice-looking man entering the apartment next door. She told him hello and introduced herself.

The man looked her dead in the face and said, "Teena, it's me. I'm just in street clothes." Her friendly neighbor, whom she had always thought was a woman, turned out to be a very charming crossdresser.

Mom was mortified! She'd already had him over for iced tea. She could handle the country music industry, but could she handle the California chaos? Not so much, especially when her baby girl was in the mix.

After only six days, my mother sent me back to Amarillo to stay with my dad and the stepmonster.

My mother might have been overwhelmed by the California lifestyle and La Jolla culture. Still, she knew an entirely different "culture" awaited me at Daddy's house, and she wouldn't leave me empty-handed and unprepared.

When I returned to my daddy's house, a box appeared in the mail. Inside were two books—*I'm OK, You're OK* by Dr. Thomas A. Harris and *Games People Play* by Dr. Eric Berne. These were two of the most foundational and popular books about transactional analysis—a method for understanding how people interact with each other and the positions they assume to conduct those interactions. Inside one of the books, I found a little note from her that said, and I'm paraphrasing, "Read these to figure out how you are going to handle what's going on over there."

Mom never came out and said it, but I knew exactly what she meant. She knew my stepmonster was playing all kinds of head games, and she knew my daddy wasn't going to protect me from them. So, those books became my summer reading. While other kids were breezing through Nancy Drew, I was neck-deep in learning how people interact and communicate. I learned how to spot manipulation, call out passive-aggressive nonsense, and hold my ground. I learned to read a room like a pro. I could sniff out a power play before the person opened their mouth. That's a pretty mature skill set for a 12-year-old.

And I'll tell you what—I didn't just read those books. I *used* them. That summer became my laboratory for human behavior. I'd go into the living room, smile at my stepmonster like the polite little girl she wanted, and immediately identify whatever manipulation she was trying to pull on me that day. Because of those books, I knew how to handle it.

Was it weird? Yes. Did it work? Absolutely.

After six weeks, Mom came back to Amarillo. She said it was because she didn't want to leave me at Daddy's with the stepmonster, but I think she wasn't prepared for the fast lifestyle in California. She was still so young—not yet 40—and didn't want to be there alone. Today, I'm grateful for the preparation she sent me in the form of those two books. Mother was wise and used her intelligence to make me smart too. By the time seventh grade rolled around, I had more emotional intelligence than most adults. I didn't know it then, but those books— *Games People Play* and *I'm OK, You're OK*—would later become secret weapons in my business arsenal.

Self-Awareness in Retrospect

I look back now, and I can see it plain as day—how much my mom gave me, even though it didn't always feel like a gift at the time. I mean, come on. What 8-year-old wants cassette tapes full of affirmations instead of a new Barbie Dreamhouse? I recognize now that she wasn't trying to raise a little girl. She didn't know how long she'd have with me, so she was trying to build a woman who could walk into a room and *own it*, whether she was 10 or 40.

Fast forward a few decades, I could walk into conference rooms on Wall Street and face down men in thousand-dollar suits who underestimated me the moment I stepped through the door. I could read them like a children's book and spot a game before the first handshake was over. I could redirect a conversation with a few words and a look. And I wasn't afraid to say the thing no one else wanted to say because I had the tools to deal with whatever came next. I wasn't just confident. I was *equipped*. I could go toe-to-toe with executives who ran billion-dollar portfolios and calmly say, "All right, boys, put your egos back in your pockets and let's talk shop." And they'd *listen*.

And let me tell you something…I didn't come by that kind of awareness by accident. That resulted from a childhood full of little experiments my mother was running. Commercials, plays, pageants, sales pitches, cassette tapes, summer reading assignments—she fed me a steady diet of confidence and provided ways to use it. I didn't know any different, and I loved it.

I think that's why I succeeded, whereas my peers sometimes stalled out. I had my version of an internal GPS built by all the stories I told, all the stages I crossed, and all the hours in the mirror with Dr. Maxwell Maltz's Confidence Building Kit. It breaks my heart to know that my sister didn't get the same tools I did. My sister spent most of her time with our grandmother, so she didn't get the cassettes. She didn't get the books. She was 16 when I was 8 and had already spent time in a residential treatment facility for drug addiction. She struggled. We had the same mom but were raised in different worlds.

My mom *tried* with my sister. She really did. But it just didn't work. It was a different time, and honestly, they were very different people. My sister was born in 1958. This would put her teenage years in the middle of the peace and love era. And maybe that whole mindset didn't do her any favors. When things got hard, she literally ran away. That was how she coped. There just wasn't a way to get through to her back then. It's hard to understand our environment back then if you weren't living in it, but there were no cell phones, no internet, and no GPS. If your kid walked out the door, they practically disappeared without a trace. Short of calling neighbors and the friends that they knew about, there wasn't much more they could do.

My mom did everything she could to get through to her. She even sent her to college, where she even got her Master's in Art Education. Me? I didn't even graduate from high school. I had to claw my way to everything I've achieved—GED, career, earning power, all of it. Nothing was handed to me.

Like I said, my mom and sister did not get along. My mom used my sister as a pawn to get what she wanted. I would love to know more about how my mom saw it, but she is not here to tell me her side. Instead, I turned to the one other person I could ask—my sister. I picked up the phone just the other day and called her because I wanted to know if Tanya felt our mother—she calls her Teenie, not "Mom" or "Mother"—ever did anything Tanya was grateful for.

"Well...she always encouraged my art," she said. "It wasn't that I was all that great. I was a so-so artist, but she always encouraged me to pursue my art."

"But you were a damn good art teacher!" I interjected. And she was. She taught art for over 30 years and was amazing at it.

"She also made sure I got my associate's degree," she continued. Tanya lived at our grandmother's house while attending Texas State Technical Institute and got her associate's degree in commercial photography. Before she could continue her education, she became pregnant by her longtime boyfriend, who would later become her husband for 47 years. It was 15 years before she could finally return to school and obtain her bachelor's degree in teaching with an art minor. She pivoted to teaching and worked her way up from there.

I don't begrudge her experience at all. She never could receive anything good from my mother, even if Mom tried to offer it. In her eyes, anything from Teenie was tainted and still is. That's just who my sister is—glass half empty.

I've always leaned the other way. I try to see the good. I don't believe my mom was ever malicious. Did she mess up? Absolutely. Was she a narcissist? Big time...but not because she wanted to hurt us. It was more like she didn't know how to be anything else. The world had revolved around her for so long that she didn't even know how to get off its axis.

Honestly, Mom didn't have a maternal bone in her body. What she *did* have was the ability to identify when someone was in trouble and be resourceful in helping them get out of it. I think it made her feel superior in some way to help someone when she could. I know she was picky about who she would help, but when she decided to help you, she was all in—as long as you did it her way.

There was always an accounting, though. She kept a mental scorecard with a tally of what she had done for you so you could be sure to repay her when she needed it later on down the road. Remember, it was still all about Teenie—her illness, her goals, her timing. We were just passengers on her roller coaster. And narcissists like her? They don't "co-" anything. Not co-parenting. Not co-working. Not co-existing. Everything is on their terms. If someone like my grandmother stepped in and said, "This isn't a good idea for Tanya," my mom's answer would be, "It'll be fine once we get there." That was always her logic— once *she* got where *she* wanted to be, the rest of us would be fine.

Except we weren't.

And I think that's what my sister resented most. My mom pulled her along for the ride when she could have stayed with my grandmother permanently. She couldn't understand why she had to endure the chaos. Instead of trying to draw me in and build something different with me, even later in life, she pushed me away too. I don't know why. Pride? Maybe. Stubbornness? Probably. It was always "I want to do it my way." Even when her way kept destroying everything in her life that was good.

My dad used the best metaphor to describe her: "Your mother likes to build sandcastles and then try to move in." I understood precisely what he meant. It was always the next book, the next song, the next idea, the next, the next, the next, the next!

And so Tanya and I grew up in the same house sometimes, but in very different worlds. My sister had the opportunity and ran from it. I had nothing and fought for everything I got. Maybe I was Mom's second chance to get it right. Either way, I'm grateful for it, even the cassette tapes and self-affirmations, because it all worked. Turns out, that's the real inheritance my mom left me.

Doing Things Differently

There are two things I want to recommend, and I can't stress them enough as this chapter comes to a close.

Get Counseling

Do not wait until things "get bad." When it comes to chronic illness, things *will* get bad—even terrible. By then, too many things have the potential to spin out of control with too many people. Depending on who and where those issues have arisen, you may be unable to reestablish some of those relationships and move forward with them.

My mother burned so many bridges, and make no mistake, she lit them up with accelerant. I am sure that if she recognized the need to burn a bridge, it must've needed burning badly. But there were times when we could have really used some help from the folks on the other side of that bridge. We were never guaranteed any, but because she had already burned the bridge, we couldn't even ask.

I don't care how strong, competent, or seasoned you think you are—getting counseling from a professional therapist shows wisdom, not weakness. If you're walking through caregiving or chronic illness, get yourself in a room with someone who can help you unpack it, whether it's just you, your partner, your kids, or your whole family.

Children who are caregivers take on decision-making way too young, long before the part of the brain that handles decision-making develops. That's how it was for me—my decision-making development was stunted. My young brain had to find ways to make decisions outside the normal neural pathways that more mature brains use. Sometimes, that resulted in me making rash decisions I had to dig myself out of later. Even so, I couldn't take a risk because I had no safety net. I couldn't afford to make too many mistakes.

I didn't start counseling until I was an adult, and it took me ten years in therapy to be able to start making decisions without second-guessing them. Because I hadn't had the time to allow my neural pathways to develop into healthy decision-making skills as a child, I had to learn it as an adult, and that was hard.

I also learned that emotions don't mean you're fragile; they indicate that you're *human*. This goes for you too. Every emotion you feel is valid—the glad, the mad, and the sad. Kids especially need help identifying and dealing with what's going on when there's trauma in their lives. I know I did.

Learn How to Communicate

I know this sounds trite, but communication is something that most people struggle with. My mother had to teach me to use the so-called "conversational ball"—the idea that when it's someone's turn to talk, you listen without interrupting—appropriately. Remember, I love to tell a good story. In elementary school, I got F's in conduct because I was too talkative. Well, I had a lot to say! Trust me—you will too.

During my second marriage, my in-laws were struck by Hurricane Katrina. They were 76 and 78 years old and trying to pick up the pieces of their damaged home, as was the entire metropolitan New Orleans area. They should've been sitting on a porch swing somewhere, sipping iced tea and enjoying retirement. And then, before we could even get them settled, my father-in-law was diagnosed with leukemia.

Now, here's where it gets interesting on the communication part. Once they had done all they could for him, treatment-wise, they elected hospice. The whole time he was in hospice, he didn't want his wife to know he was dying, and she didn't want him to know that *she knew* he was dying. The two of them danced around each other while I ran back and forth between them, coordinating hospice, managing the details, and holding the whole thing together. We had the same conversations repeatedly.

I'd walk into the bedroom where he rested and say, "Don't you think she knows?"

"Well…" He'd look at me blankly.

"Come on. You really think you're hiding this from her? She *knows*," I told him, sighing.

Then I'd wander into the kitchen with her and say, "Don't you think he *knows* you know?"

She'd shake her head. "He believes I think he's gonna live forever."

And I'd say, "Oh, Loretta. I love you. But no. He knows. And you *know* he knows. Now y'all need to talk."

Multiply that moment right there by *hundreds*. I've done this song and dance so many times with families, clients, and couples to gently (or not-so-gently) push them toward the conversations they're scared to have.

Being scared isn't a good enough reason to pretend something isn't happening.

That doesn't protect anyone. It just isolates everybody. You have to *say the thing*. You have to name what's going on.

One of the most essential pieces of advice I can give you is that it is vital to learn how to talk to each other about everything—logistics, feelings, grief, and love. Whatever is going on, keep the lines of communication open.

When I entered the financial planning business, people asked me what I would specialize in. The thing is, most insurance products available cover events that may or may not happen, depending on various circumstances.

Retirement? Maybe you make it to retirement, or perhaps you don't.

Disability? It's not a given, and I pray you'll never experience being disabled.

Long-term care? If you live long enough, you are more than likely to have a chronic illness or need long-term care. But I mean, that's still not a sure thing.

But you know what's *not* optional? Death. Everyone on the planet will eventually die, so I decided to focus my attention on life insurance products. The only question I had to gain consent on when speaking with people was, "Do you care enough about those who depend on you for financial support to plan for when you exit this earth so they at least won't immediately have to change their standard of living?"

Make that your starting line. If you love somebody, then you've got a reason to talk. Everything else—money, health, time—can get figured out if you just keep talking. How can I talk about all this stuff without flinching? Because I grew up with it. My mom was dying my whole life, and she didn't try to hide it. It was part of the backdrop of our lives and the air we breathed. Because of that, it never became a dirty secret or a ticking time bomb. It was just the truth—a hard one, but a livable one.

So that's what I want for you too. Don't pretend the hard stuff isn't real. Don't shove it down and smile through it. Speak it. Name it. Look it in the eye because you can survive anything if you stop pretending and start preparing.

When I became a mother, I knew I wanted to do things differently based on what I had gone through. I'd been asked to carry way too much, way too soon. So, I was very mindful of what I handed to my kids. They had chores, sure—but they also had space just to be kids. They didn't have to make their breakfast at 5 years old or emotionally babysit me. I wanted them to grow up feeling supported while also being responsible. I even allowed them to have an opinion! Did I always go along with their views? I considered their perspectives, but ultimately, as the parent, I made the decisions, and they knew it.

I also taught them early how to handle money, advocate for themselves, and name what they were feeling and not be ashamed of it. We talked about hard things. We laughed, cried when needed, and told the truth—even when it was uncomfortable. Because I knew firsthand that stuffing things down only turns them into landmines later, I wanted my children to have tools, not trauma.

My mother didn't always know how to love maternally, but she *did* instill in me the belief that with the right tools and resources, I could probably do anything I wanted. This is why I want to encourage you to take action now. Don't wait. Don't tough things out. Don't shove things down and hope they'll go away. Call a counselor and learn how to sit down with your people and say, "Hey. This is hard. Let's figure it out together." You deserve that. And the people who love you deserve it too.

Chapter 6

Using the Skills She Taught Me

When people ask me how often my mom got sick, I tell them, "She was always sick."

And I mean that. Even before I was 5 years old, my mother's illness wasn't just an occasional thing. It wasn't like we went to the doctor now and then. We were constantly—*constantly*—at the doctor's office or the hospital. I'm talking two or three times a week, easily.

"Get in the car," she'd say when she picked me up from school. "I gotta get to Dr. Dine's office before it closes so I can get my bloodwork done."

And off we'd go, speeding through town, trying to beat the clock before the lab shut down for the day. If you grew up in a normal household, maybe that sounds wild. To me, that was just another day.

Her white blood cell count was our barometer. If it spiked, that meant an infection, which meant she was going to be spending some time in the hospital again. I didn't know it back then, but infection is what eventually ends the lives of people with Crohn's disease. The disease itself won't kill you, but the infection your body can't fight off because your immune system is shot to hell will. Crohn's lived in the background of everything we did. I was always aware of it, even if I didn't always talk about it.

Life in the Waiting Room

The only real treatment available when she'd have flare-ups was prednisone, which was the answer to almost anything that was inflamed and required a sustained treatment to reduce that inflammation. With Crohn's, the intestine can easily become inflamed, swollen, and sometimes ulcerated. That inflammation, due to a bad flare, can also create narrowed areas called strictures or fistulas—tunnels that form between the bowel and other organs or skin. When the prednisone quit working and a flareup got bad enough that it had to be dealt with, the only other option was to resect, or cut out, part of her small intestine. And that was a problem because the small intestine is responsible for digesting food and absorbing the nutrients your body needs from food.

Once Mom's surgeon started cutting pieces of her small intestine out—something that only happened when there was no other option—my mom's body lost the ability to absorb nutrients properly and digest food. Instead, food rushed straight to her colon, undigested, from where it would be quickly expelled.

She dealt with a lot of pain and inflammation, and there were a lot of foods she just couldn't eat. On top of all that, she had pernicious anemia because she couldn't absorb any nutrition from the foods she *could* eat. She had to take B12 shots every month and suffered from debilitating exhaustion. I can't remember a single day when she didn't take at least two or three naps just to make it through.

Even if she hadn't been so exhausted all the time, she still didn't get out much because she was allergic to the sun. She'd had a sunstroke as a teenager, and doctors think that might've been the trigger that activated her Crohn's disease. She couldn't handle heat or light. And because she couldn't be out in the sun, she didn't come to many school events. In fact, she didn't come to *any* school events.

And it wasn't just Crohn's. She had kidney stones all the time—bad ones. The kind that would've sent most people straight to surgery. But my mom? She passed them naturally. Every time. Because after the kind of pain she lived with day in and day out, a kidney stone didn't seem like that big of a deal.

The crazy thing was, she looked fine. That was her superpower…and her curse. When the nursing homes started turning her down later in life, we couldn't figure out why. Then we realized—she was dressing up for the interviews, taking a pain pill, and putting on makeup so that she didn't look or act sick. And when you don't look or act sick, people don't believe you are.

That's the thing about chronic illness—it doesn't just chip away at the person who has it. It eats away at everything around them too. Time. Energy. Family. Possibility. For example, we didn't go out to eat. My mother couldn't eat restaurant food because she could never be sure what was in it. Even just black pepper could make her miserable. So we stayed close to home, eating supper at my grandmother's house almost every night. We didn't have the money to eat out anyway.

To me, it wasn't tragic. I was just an easy-going, happy kid. This was my life, and I was going to make the best of it. It was kind of like living in the eye of a storm that never let up. You got good at checking the wind, watching the clouds, and bracing for whatever came next. Because you knew it *would* come, and you'd better be ready.

So when people say, "Your mom was sick a lot, huh?" I nod and smile. But what I really want to say is, "You have no idea!"

We lived in the waiting room of the doctor's office, the hospital, and life. I learned to function in that space because I didn't know anything different. But it wouldn't be long before life threw me into a situation where I *was* thrown for a loop. I was about to get knocked around pretty good, and I was going to need every ounce of confidence my mom and Dr. Maxwell Maltz (the guy on the cassette tapes) had worked so hard to build in me.

It was time to find out just how much those tools were worth.

The First Test

Junior high was a defining season for me—especially eighth grade. If you'd asked me at the beginning of the year, I'd have told you I was doing great. I loved junior high. In fact, if you plucked out just those junior high years—everything *except* what happened at the end of eighth grade—I'd tell you they were some of the best years of my life. Which, looking back, is kind of heartbreaking. Isn't it sad when your life peaks years before you even have boobs?

I was a confident, popular young teenager. One thing I always had going for me was that I had a lot of friends. I wasn't the prettiest girl in school, but I was funny, well-liked, and outgoing. Thanks to all the "mirror time" I'd clocked with Dr. Maxwell Maltz's cassette tapes, I was pretty dang sure of myself. I knew how to walk into a room, command attention, and win people over. Plus, at just 100 pounds, I was the perfect size to be a flyer—the cheerleader who did jumps and stunts from the top of the pyramid. I'd earned that confidence. My mother made damn sure of it.

And then came cheerleader tryouts.

My friend Lisa, who was in the grade ahead of me, was aging out of the squad and moving on to high school. Same with another girl. That meant there were two open spots on the cheerleading team—and everyone said one of them had my name on it. I'd put in the work. I learned the routines, smiled the smile, and nailed the tryout. And when I say I nailed it, I mean I *nailed it*. Even the people running the tryouts pulled me aside and told me, "It's yours. It's yours, Shelly."

It felt like something good was finally happening. Something was finally going *my* way. And the best part? My mom came to the assembly. For once, she actually *came*. She'd made it to the school auditorium that morning at 11 a.m.—despite her illness, despite the sun allergy, despite everything. That was rare. That was huge.

The first name was called. It wasn't mine.

That's okay. They'll call me next.

But they didn't. They called a girl named Alane.

Now listen. When I tell you hardly anyone knew who Alane was, I'm not being catty. We'd gone to school together since third grade, but hardly anyone in the breezeway recognized her name, at least in eighth grade. Everyone was looking around, thinking another girl named Elaine had somehow tried out when no one noticed.

Even though it broke my heart that I hadn't made the squad, I spoke up to make sure she was acknowledged.

"No, not *E*laine, *A*lane. Alane Snyder!" Alane was my friend.

I kept it together, but barely. A day or two later, I was pulled aside afterward by someone who had been involved in the counting of the votes, and they said, "I need you to know something. You *did* have the most votes. The student votes came in, and you won. But the cheerleading coach swapped your name out for Alane's because the coach doesn't like you, and she was also afraid your parents couldn't afford it."

My not making the cheerleading team wasn't about talent, leadership, popularity, or effort. It boiled down to my life's circumstances.

I don't remember what Alane's dad did, but her mom was a teacher, and they lived in a ritzy neighborhood with a tennis court in the backyard. Meanwhile, I lived in a not-so-great neighborhood in a house my dad had bought for $10,000 ten years before. I was glad to have a house, but it was so run down and dilapidated that when someone gave me a ride home, I had them drop me off around the corner so they didn't see where I lived.

The teachers and coaches knew about my mom's illness, and they were aware of where I lived. They saw how I was often late and missed days of school. They assumed we couldn't pay for the uniform or the travel or whatever else they thought cheerleaders needed, so they decided *for* me. No conversation. No option to say, "My dad can cover it." Just...disqualified.

The worst part about the whole thing was that this assembly was the *one* thing my mom came to. She'd dragged her tired, hurting body out of the house and into a sunny courtyard on a spring afternoon and braved the emotional and physical toll it would take on her to be surrounded by teenagers—to see me shine.

But I didn't. Not because I hadn't earned it, but because someone else decided I didn't belong. It was a gut punch. For the first time, I saw how the world really worked, and I realized I didn't come from the right side of the tracks. That was my first taste of what it felt like to be disenfranchised—blocked from opportunity because of who I was and where I was from. It made me realize just how often the world would try to make decisions for me based on the parts of my story I couldn't control.

I learned something big that day. I learned that if you're not in the room when decisions are made—and especially if people assume you don't have money—you'd better believe they'll write you off before you ever get a chance to prove them wrong. That's exactly what was done to me.

I wasn't mad at Alane. I had known her since I was in third grade. I'd spent the night over at her house and she at mine many, many times over the previous decade, and I still see her to this day. I was mad at the system and the adults who thought they were protecting me from embarrassment by choosing to embarrass me. I was mad at the people who thought they were helping when really, they were just proving that no matter how much confidence my mother had instilled in me, the world would still find a way to shove me back into my "place."

The sad thing was that my mom and I might not have had much money, but my dad did. He would have bought that uniform or whatever was needed in a heartbeat, but they never gave me the chance to even ask. They just assumed.

So I went home, and I cried. Who wouldn't? Then I dried my tears and squared my shoulders. I still had the confidence tools my mother gave me, and whether the school staff wanted me on the cheer squad or not, I knew exactly what kind of girl I was. I may not have been a cheerleader, but I was still a leader, a scrapper, and a fighter.

Class Drama Becomes Trauma

After the cheerleader fiasco, life went on. It wasn't easy knowing the one thing that I'd worked extremely hard for—joining the cheerleading squad—had been yanked away because someone decided I wasn't the "right kind of girl." But I still had my friends. I still had my confidence—shaken, sure, but not broken.

At least, not yet.

Eighth grade started off as one of the best years of my life. Our class at Crockett Junior High was close. Weirdly close. Unlike most junior highs, where the boys sat on one side of the cafeteria and the girls sat on the other, we all sat together. Nobody could tell who was dating whom. We were just *us*—a tight-knit, messy little family. Even the school principal said he'd never seen a class that close.

But things unraveled quickly for me that spring, and—as happens with most junior high drama—it started with something stupid. One of the boys in our group—I'll call him Harvey—decided it would be funny to tell another girl in our math class, Catherine, that I had shared with everyone that she had started her period.

I mean...seriously?

In eighth grade, that kind of thing can get blown out of proportion fast. It shouldn't, but it does. And even though it sounds ridiculous now, at the time, it felt like a big deal.

I was oblivious to the drama until Catherine's friend Cindy marched up to me in a huff in the hallway between classes.

"Did you tell Harvey that Catherine started her period?"

"What?" I blinked at her. "No. I didn't even know she had."

"Well," Cindy said, "she didn't."

"Well, I didn't even know that," I responded. "Whatever." And that was that. With my mom's chronic illness, I'd never really been much for that kind of small-time petty bullshit. I figured it was just a dumb misunderstanding, shrugged to myself, and went on with my day.

But when I got to my next class, things were…off. That's when I knew something wasn't right. No one would look at me or talk to me. People were whispering and avoiding me, and for a kid whose friends had always surrounded them, that wasn't normal.

Then, after lunch, someone handed me a note. From the outside, it looked like any other note that got passed in the hall or the classroom. The note was folded over into a rectangle with the jagged edges from the spiral ring on one side of the fold.

But it wasn't your typical, "Do you like Chris? Circle yes or no" kind of note. It was a direct hit. When I opened it, I found my school picture inside. My eyes had been sliced with a protractor and crossed out. The words "Eat shit and die" were scribbled on the paper in permanent marker.

And it was signed by ten people. I recognized the names of friends and classmates I'd always laughed with, shared snacks with, and yes, passed notes with. I scanned the list, and when I got to the final signature, I realized it wasn't real.

Oh, the note was real, and my crossed out school photo was real, but the last signature wasn't. I *knew* that signature, and whoever had forged it did a horrible job. There at the bottom was Goose, the name of my elementary school crush—a boy I'd been friends with since forever. He was sweet and funny and kind—the kind of boy who made you believe boys might not all be jerks.

I knew it wasn't really him. I also knew they picked his name on purpose because they knew it would hurt. I took the note straight to Goose.

"Did you sign this?" I shoved the note under his nose while he changed his books out at his locker for his next class.

He glanced down at it, then did a double take and gave it a closer look. "What is this? No. No, Shelly. I don't even know what this is."

He was angry and embarrassed. He asked me to give it to him so he could get to the bottom of it, but I didn't. I took it to the assistant principal instead, and that was the beginning of the end for me that school year. To his credit, the assistant principal took the note seriously. He pulled every kid whose name was on that note into his office, and while he read them the riot act, I went home. I'd had about all I could take for one day.

Unfortunately, the damage was already done.

That afternoon, the phone started ringing at home. The same kids who signed the note were now threatening me from the pay phone in the hallway outside the school office. When my mom called the school to report it, the assistant principal— bless his heart—tried to help. He called another round of meetings, this time with the students and their parents.

Did that actually change anything?

Nope. Not a thing. These kids kept calling at all hours of the day and night. After several days of this, my mom could see it wearing on me. She called the school again and talked to the same assistant principal.

"I can get them to quit making the calls during the day," he said. "I can do that. What I can't control is what's happening at night." After calling all the parents and students in again, the daytime calls stopped. But the whispering and forced isolation didn't. And night after night, the calls continued.

I wasn't completely alone. The boys—the ones who'd always had my back—saw what was happening, and they weren't okay with it. They were sick of the unfair way I was being treated, especially since everybody knew I hadn't done anything wrong. They knew they couldn't do anything about the way the girls in my class were acting, but they could have an impact on the other guys.

During those two weeks of living hell at school, I decided to head down to the ninth graders' football game. They were playing the eighth graders. I could hear the pep band playing, and I was lonely. I also thought maybe I was making a mountain out of a molehill. I really wanted to get out of the house, and the walk to the football field was just four blocks. Unfortunately, the minute I walked through the gates of the field, Harvey spotted me.

"Oooooh, Shelly's here!" he called out in a mocking voice. "Everybody leave! Everybody leave!"

That was all it took for some of my guy friends to step in. My really good guy friend Mickey, his best friend Don, Tommy, and a few others made eye contact with each other, then followed Harvey into the men's bathroom. They were all friends of his, so when he noticed them behind him, he turned around, laughing.

"Hey guys, did you see who's here…"

SLAM! Mickey and Tommy shoved Harvey up against the wall. "Dude, you better lay off," Mickey said as he held Harvey against the wall. "If the girls want to do this, that's on them. But you started it, and you're going to end your part in it now."

Mickey called me that night to tell me what happened. They wanted me to know that the guys were on my side and that they had my back. I thanked him. I needed to hear that, and Harvey did back off after that. He didn't try to stop the way the girls were treating me, but he quit egging them on.

The wounds still felt fresh, though, and the effortless trust I'd once had in my friends was gone. That experience was my first lesson in what it means to be targeted, discarded, and betrayed by the people who once called you a friend.

I was a social kid who thrived on connections. I wasn't just popular—I was plugged in. I'd never known what it was like to be *excluded* by my peers. And let me tell you something—when you go from belonging to being erased, it's a special kind of hell. Even my lifelong best friend turned her back on me. By the second week, my mom could tell something was breaking inside me. I wasn't eating. I wasn't talking. I didn't want to go to school, and that had *never* happened before.

So we pulled me out of Crockett Junior High because she was concerned about my mental health.

Now, keep in mind—this was during a gas crisis, and we were poor. We drove old cop cars that my Great-Uncle Cotton could get us for dirt cheap from his used car lot. They had great engines and terrible gas mileage. So when my mom arranged for me to transfer to another junior high across town—Fannin—it was a *huge* deal because those were the days when we could barely afford a trip around the block, much less a trip halfway across town.

But she did it for me. Things were better at the new school. I knew a few people there already, and I finished out the last six weeks of the school year without drama.

That summer, though, was the loneliest of my life. I didn't want to live. I didn't say that out loud at the time, but it was true. From March to August, I was barely hanging on. You know what kept me from breaking? The confidence my mom had built in me. Yes, there were cracks in the foundation, but I was still standing.

Returning With My Head—and Fists—Held High

When school started that fall, I returned to Crockett Junior High. We couldn't afford the gas it would take to drive back and forth to Fannin every day. It wasn't easy walking back through the doors. I managed to lie low all morning, quietly going from class to class. But there was no avoiding the one place I knew was going to be all eyes on me—the cafeteria at lunch.

I'd been across enough pageant stages that I could fake a confident walk with the best of them, and that's what I did. I walked into that cafeteria on my first day back with my head high and nerves in knots. I could tell a lot of people were surprised to see me. After all, this was back in the late '70s, before the internet and social media made everybody's business public knowledge. When I disappeared from school, I was just gone. Nobody really knew where I went, and nobody expected me when I came back. It didn't take long for them to roll out the welcome mat.

Catherine and Cindy walked up to me, and Cindy opened her mouth first.

"I heard through the grapevine that you said that if we do anything to piss you off, you're gonna kick our ass."

Oh no. I was *not* going right back into the same drama I'd left behind. I knew that how I reacted in that moment would set the tone for the way the rest—or at least the first part—of my ninth-grade year went, and I'd had enough. I grabbed Cindy by the front of her shirt, pulled her in close, and said, "Yeah, I'm going to kick your ass and anybody else's who tries to mess with me because I'm done with this."

And I *meant* it. After that, I fought. I fought physically when it was required and verbally quite regularly. I was maybe 100 pounds soaking wet, but I threw punches like someone twice my size. I became a scrapper, not because I wanted to, but because in order to avoid going back to being invisible, I felt like I had to.

Now, I don't recommend taking this approach, but I don't regret it either. Sometimes the only way to stop the bleeding is to swing back, so I swung. I'd lived through two weeks of hell in my eighth-grade year, alternately being ignored at school and harassed over the phone at home. And I'd survived a long, lonely summer filled with silence from the people I had called my friends. I wasn't going back to that. If I had to fight to be seen and taken seriously, so be it.

Building With Broken Bricks

Looking back now, I know what saved me. It wasn't the assistant principal or the new school or even the boys who told Harvey to lay off. What saved me were the confidence-building tools my mother gave me *before* my eighth-grade year. By that time, I already had a deep, come-hell-or-high-water sense that I mattered. I believed I was a person who was worth something. If I hadn't had that, I don't think I'd be here today.

What happened in eighth grade broke something inside me and that summer nearly crushed me. But if you had seen me the fall of my ninth-grade year—walking back into Crockett with my chin high and my fists ready—you'd probably have said, "She's fine."

I wasn't fine, but I'd built armor over that summer—thick, heavy stuff made from every cruel word, every silent lunch table, and every phone call meant to scare me. It did what armor does—it kept people out. But it also kept me in. I became the girl who smiled but stayed guarded. I was still quick with a joke but quicker with a comeback, and I wasn't afraid to throw hands if I had to.

Yet I didn't fall apart the way some kids might have. I didn't start drinking or flunk out or disappear. I still went to school. I still made decent grades. I still smiled. I still showed up. I didn't look like I was struggling, and that's exactly how I fell through the cracks.

No one thought to look closer. No one asked, "Shelly, are you okay?" I wasn't okay, but I wasn't *obviously* struggling either. I just kind of...bumped along quietly with a smile on my face. My IQ in the seventh grade was 119, but my report card was full of C's. I probably had undiagnosed dyslexia, and algebra might as well have been ancient Greek. But I looked like I was "fine," and kids who looked "fine" don't get flagged.

Kids who grow up in chaos get really, really good at hiding. I learned how to mask, how to blend, and how to play the role of the competent child so well that the adults around me forgot to check beneath the surface. I was emotionally intelligent and funny with a big personality, so nobody noticed when the girl with all that personality started building walls.

If I hadn't had that confidence kit at age 8...

If I hadn't had the mirror, the affirmations, and the books about transactional analysis...

If my mom hadn't seen something in me and poured into that part of me *on purpose*...

I don't think I would've made it. As it was, I was barely hanging on by a thread. So are a lot of the kids that nobody is looking out for. When you're not the squeaky wheel or the one blowing up in class, running away, or stealing cars, people don't think to question how things are really going. You just keep showing up, smiling, and slowly shutting down.

I know now that most kids in my situation wouldn't have survived that season the way I did. And many of them, including some of my old classmates, didn't. Some turned to drugs, some got pregnant, and some checked out completely. I hung in there, though, because I was equipped with just enough belief in myself to say, "This isn't where my story ends."

I didn't get smooth, pretty materials to create my life with. I didn't get a strong foundation. I just picked up the broken bricks life served me and got to work. Whatever I could salvage—scraps of encouragement, a few decent teachers, a handful of loyal friends, and those worn-out cassette tapes—I took it all and kept building.

Doing Things Differently

The hardest part about what happened to me during eighth grade was that nobody *really* saw it. Not the teachers. Not the school counselors. Not even the adults who were supposed to be paying attention. I didn't walk around looking like a kid in crisis. I wasn't disheveled. I wasn't failing my classes. I wasn't shoplifting or setting fires or screaming for help in the obvious ways.

I was doing okay enough that nobody stopped to look closer. Because I didn't "look the part," nobody thought I needed help. I was smiling, happy, and making jokes. That's how kids like me fall through the cracks. You want to know what it really looks like when a kid is in trouble? Sometimes it looks like the kid who never asks for anything. Sometimes it looks like the kid who makes everybody laugh. And sometimes it looks like the kid who seems to be "handling it."

Make no mistake. Kids like me make it so easy for the world to think we're okay. We're good at doing that because we've had no other choice. Even though most adults want to help, they're looking for the wrong signs. They're looking for the kid who lashes out, not the one who disappears behind a bright smile and a quick comeback.

So let me say this as plainly as I can—don't let the exterior fool you. If you're a teacher, coach, counselor, church leader— heck, even a neighbor—look again. Don't assume that just because a kid seems fine, they are. If you're in a position to check in, *check in*. Sit down with them and ask real questions. Get curious about their lives. Behind every high-functioning, overperforming, always-helpful kid, there's a story. Sometimes that story is full of trauma that they've never spoken out loud.

I've volunteered in middle schools, working with school counselors who are so overworked and assigned hundreds of students each. They can maybe help two or three a year with the time and resources they have, and that's not enough. There are way too many kids out there who are carrying too much and doing the best they can to hold life together. Yet the ones who need the most support are often the ones we notice the least.

I know because I was one of them. I made it, but barely. If it wasn't for the confidence my mother instilled in me and the toolkit she handed me *before* everything hit the fan, things could have been very different for me. If you take nothing else from this chapter, take this: Look for the kids who hide their struggles well.

Look for the ones who smile a little too hard, never ask for anything, and always seem "fine." Ask them real questions, and show up in their lives on purpose. When you get the chance to speak life into them, don't hold back. Because you never know when your words might be the first thing that makes them believe they can actually make it through whatever they're in.

Chapter 7

Let's Take a (Mental) Break

Y ou could say I grew up in the glow of my mother's desk lamp as she pounded out stories and interviews on her typewriter late into the night.

Long after most moms had gone to bed, mine was just getting started with her day. She'd be hunched over her typewriter—clicking away at an article, a ghostwriting project, or some piece for *Texas Monthly* or a local newsletter. I'd fall asleep to the rhythm of her tapping the keys with purpose, and if I woke up in the middle of the night, she'd still be at it, chasing down whatever wild idea had taken hold of her.

Her unorthodox schedule meant that she didn't come to my school activities. Thankfully, I wasn't athletic anyway. The only time I tried out for a sport was when a friend asked me to, and let's just say I was really good at riding the bench. But if I was out and about at night, my friends and I always had a ride home. The other parents loved this because they didn't have to get out of bed in the middle of the night to play chauffeur.

That was the trade-off. She wasn't the mom in the bleachers, but she *was* the one up late, willing to drive across town to pick up a carload of girls after the movies or take us from one teen club to another when no other parent wanted to. I had a lot of friends, and these friends thought my mom was cool—hippie cool, but without the drugs. She played guitar and read tarot cards, something she later quit doing because she said God told her to "knock it off" or she was going to die. Even today, classmates at my school reunions ask me about her.

"Oh, Shelly! How is your mother? She was so cool!"

She wasn't that way with only my friends and me. She was the mom who rescued my sister's friends when they'd partied too hard. I remember a time we picked up my sister, Tanya, and one of her friends. The friend had overdosed while huffing paint. I know my mom insisted on calling the kid's parents, and he didn't want to do that, so he jumped out of the car on the way to the hospital.

She operated with what looked like grace on the outside, but underneath it all—she was unraveling.

Problems With Prednisone

Doctors had put my mom on prednisone after her hospital stay when I was 5, and it was the only thing keeping her from having another resection. For someone with Crohn's, that usually means a section that's been so inflamed, scarred, or narrowed that food can't pass through easily anymore—or at all. A resection gave her some relief and a window of time to rebuild strength, but it's not a cure. Crohn's doesn't just go away, and a person only has so much intestine to resect. I've always referred to Crohn's disease as a chronic pain in the ass that you can't die from, but every day you'll wish you could.

Prednisone kept her body functioning and the Crohn's flare-ups to a minimum—and believe me, flare-ups are not fun. A Crohn's flare-up can feel like your body just decides to go to war with itself, and you're the battlefield. It can start slow, like a nagging stomach ache that won't quit. Or it can hit out of nowhere with sharp pain and cramping so bad it takes your breath away. You can't eat. Or you try, and it runs right through you. The fatigue sets in, too, and it's not just "I need a nap" tired. It's the kind of tired that makes you feel like you're climbing a mountain instead of brushing your teeth.

So for Mom, prednisone was a lifesaver. The problem was, the longer she was on it, the more she needed because her body built up a tolerance to it. She started out with 10 mg a day, then 20 mg, then 30 mg, but she'd long since maxed out at 65 mg daily. The doctors knew steroids like prednisone could cause some serious psychotic issues, so they'd put her on it, then take her back off, over and over again—all while hoping to keep the psychological effects to a minimum.

It *was* affecting her, though. Back then, I knew nothing different. To me, she'd always been unpredictable and had struggled with paranoia for as long as I could remember. Even when I was little, she would send me through the house to check for intruders whenever we'd been away because she was convinced someone had gotten into the house while we were gone, even if it had only been for two hours.

Just so you understand, her rationale was that I was young and could run, while she was sick and would never be able to get out of the house in time. Talk about a harrowing childhood experience. I brought this memory up to her years later when she was in the nursing home.

"I did not! You're lying!" she accused me.

"No, I'm not lying!" I recoiled and snapped back. "Call my sister. You made her do it too!"

"Well, if I did that—and I'm not admitting that I did—that would make me a terrible mother."

"Well, it is what it is," I responded.

Prednisone kept her on edge all the time. For example, she'd been trying to quit smoking for years. Sometimes she'd go to extreme measures to keep her quitting streak going.

"Take these keys," she'd say, shoving them at me. "I'm trying to quit smoking. Don't let me have them, no matter what I say to you. Hide them."

So I'd go hide them. After all, that's what she said she wanted, right?

Yet four hours later, she was slamming me up against the wall, yelling, "Where are the keys?"

"You told me not to give them to you!"

"I didn't mean it. Give them to me now!"

So I'd go get the keys and hand them over. I was a kid. What else could I do? And off she'd go to get her cigarettes. By the time she came back, she'd have calmed down.

"I'm sorry," she'd say. "I'm sorry. I shouldn't have done that."

After a while, I recognized the cycle that kept happening. So, I quit taking the keys and told her I wasn't going to be responsible for that anymore.

In Texas in the 1970s, you could apply for a hardship driver's license, sometimes called a minor restricted driver's license, if there was a family hardship or medical necessity. Yep, that was us. By the time I was 15, I'd earned my hardship driver's license and was able to drive myself wherever I needed to go. It was great to be able to get myself to school or to babysitting jobs, but when I returned home, I never knew what kind of mother I was going to find. One minute she'd be bright, funny, and full of fire. The next moment she was screaming at me and throwing things around.

To most people, that would sound absurd. To me, it just sounded like a Tuesday. Although my mother was better physically on prednisone, one of the biggest side effects she experienced was that she couldn't sleep. Hence the late-night writing sessions. She did some of her best writing in the middle of the night. When she was in the middle of a project, she was brilliant. When she was able to work, it paid well…kind of. She was really bad with money, and she knew it. So instead of getting paid in cash, she'd ask for things like new carpet or a carport for the house. I mean, that worked to meet a need, I guess. We couldn't eat new carpet or a new carport, but I do understand what she was trying to do. She knew she could never save up $5,000 or $10,000 to pay for anything, so when one of her ghostwriting gigs would pay her a handsome sum, she would never let that large sum touch her hands until the big items she had earmarked as needs were taken care of.

When you grow up in that kind of environment, you don't react to the craziness. You don't ask questions, and you don't sound the alarm. You just keep going about your daily life. Years later, I came across psychologist John Bradshaw's work, and something he said in his first book, *Bradshaw On: The Family, A New Way of Creating Solid Self-Esteem*, stuck with me. He talked about how kids from traumatic homes learn to normalize things that would be obvious and alarming to others.

He described how, for most people, if a bag of trash suddenly fell from the sky in front of them, they'd stop, look up, and try to figure out what just happened. But kids like me? We just step around the trash and keep going because it seems like trash falling out of the sky all the time is normal. That was my whole life. The paranoia, the outbursts, the uninhibited buying habits—I didn't question any of it. I just adapted and adjusted.

I'll never forget when my mom got it in her head that the CNN jingle was a divine signal that she needed to buy something. Whenever that deep, dramatic tone they used at the top of the hour came on, "Dun-dun-dun-dunnnn," she believed she needed to change the channel to QVC and buy whatever was on.

I want to point out that there were no remotes back then. You had to get up and turn the dial physically. So every hour, like clockwork, she'd hear that CNN jingle, pop up from her chair, and twist the knob over to QVC. God forbid we had breaking news! I didn't think much of it at first—this was just more of Mom being…Mom. But then stuff started showing up at the house.

At first, it was a Ginsu knife set. Okay, fine, maybe we needed knives. But then a second set showed up, and a third. Suddenly we had three woks, too, and *nobody* needs that much stir-fry.

I remember asking her, "Where is all this coming from?" And she just looked at me, totally matter-of-fact, and said, "I think God wants me to buy these." That's when it hit me—she really believed it. She believed that when CNN played its theme music, it was some kind of divine cue, and QVC was the message she was supposed to receive.

Then I discovered that Fingerhut—the mail-order catalog that sold cheap knickknacks—had given her a line of credit. I swear, Fingerhut would give a line of credit to a raccoon with a mailing address! Except for the (newly increased) $400 a month in child support my dad gave us, we were broke. You better believe everyone got a wok or a knife set for Christmas that year.

I didn't know the term "steroid psychosis" at the time, but I do now. Back then, I just thought…*trash is falling from the sky again. Step around it, Shelly. Keep walking.*

But the night I had to check my mother into a psychiatric hospital when I was only 15—that was the night the trash hit me square in the chest. And for the first time, I couldn't just step over it. I had to deal with it.

Fire and Brimstone in the Corner

There was always a low-level hum of instability in our house, but the year my mom had her full-blown psychotic break, the volume got cranked all the way up.

Looking back, the signs were there. I just didn't know enough about the effects of long-term steroid use. At this point, she'd been on 65 mg of prednisone a day for three years straight. It kept her body out of the hospital, but it was tearing her mind to shreds. I thought the hallucinations, the paranoia, the outbursts—that was just my mom being sick. I didn't know it was steroid psychosis.

Then one day, she told me she smelled fire and brimstone in the corner of the den. That was one of the first big red flags. That same week, my mom's sister was in town, and she and Grandmother came to visit every day for several days. I mentioned it to my grandmother in passing, as if it were just another Tuesday.

"Hey, Mom says she smells fire and brimstone in the den."

But instead of brushing it off like I expected, she and my aunt got really quiet.

"Yeah," they said. "She told us that too." And that's when I realized they were worried. And if *they* were worried, my mom and I were probably in trouble.

I came home from school on the second day of their visit and found all three of them—my mom, my aunt, and my grandmother—sitting on the couch. My grandmother had some soup and was trying to feed it to my mom. You could cut the tension with a Ginsu knife.

"What's going on?" I asked.

"She won't eat," Grandmother said.

"Well, is she hungry?"

"No, I'm not," Mom answered for herself.

"Well then, she's not hungry." I shrugged and went down the hall to my room. Grandmother followed me.

"She won't eat for us, Shelly," she told me. "She thinks your aunt and I put poison in her food, but she says she'll eat for you."

That's when it shifted for me. This wasn't just Mom being eccentric or unpredictable. This was something else. Something worse. And I was the only person she trusted. I went out to the living room and fed her the soup, then went back to my bedroom and called the boy I was dating at the time.

"Hey, what's going on?" he asked.

"Oh, I was just feeding my mom. She won't eat for my aunt or my grandmother. She thinks they're trying to poison her."

"Wait, what? That's crazy! And you're just sitting here talking on the phone? Is your door locked?"

"Ummmm, no."

"Don't you think it should be?" he asked. Trash was falling from the sky around me. He could see it, but I was still trying to step around it.

Eventually, it reached a point where we had no choice but to do something drastic. On the fifth day of their visit, Grandma and my aunt came to me and said, "She hasn't eaten for three days, and she won't let us take her to the hospital. But she says she'll go with you." So we got in the car, and I drove my own mother to the ER at Northwest Hospital. My hardship license had never felt more appropriately named than in that moment.

When we got there, they took her back immediately. My grandmother went with her, and my aunt and I sat out in the waiting area. They saw that Mom was having steroid psychosis and knew that once they took her off the medication, she would be golden. To get her the help she needed, they wanted her to be admitted to the Pavilion, our local psychiatric hospital, where she could receive care under the family's directive.

That's about when the door to the exam room opened, and she saw me. Suddenly, she calmed down, quit arguing, and said, "I'll go if my daughter takes me." And that was it. I became the one responsible for delivering her to the psychiatric hospital. She finally agreed she would go.

I remember that 15-minute drive as if it were happening in slow motion. She was quiet the whole way—fragile but alert. I kept thinking, *What if she turns on me? What if she suddenly decides I'm not safe either?* Because when someone's that far gone, you don't know what their mind is going to do next. I can't believe they just sent us off together in that car alone. Thankfully, we made it.

I'm not sure how, but somehow my aunt and grandmother arrived before Mom and I did. Grandmother was already filling out paperwork. I sat Mom down next to my grandmother. Almost immediately, Grandmother approached me and said, "She won't let me sign the paperwork because she still thinks Terri and I are trying to kill her. And because she seems lucid right now, they're not willing to use a physician's certificate to commit her, which would only require them to do a 72-hour hold on her."

I stepped in. I'd been legally emancipated for two years (more about that in the next chapter). If she was going to get the help she needed and she refused to do it for herself, it was up to me. I'd have to have her admitted. I sat down in front of the paperwork Grandmother had started and continued filling it out as I talked to my mother.

"Mom, you're not thinking correctly. These people will help you." I reminded her of what had been going on lately with the woks and Ginsu knives and the fire and brimstone. "I can't have you come back to the house with me like that. Could you at least let these people put you in for a couple of days? That's all they have to do."

As I held the pen over the signature field to have her admitted, in a moment I will never forget, Mom reached over and put her hand on mine. She looked at the intake nurse, then at the paperwork in front of me.

"Wait a minute," she asked. "If she signs this, does that mean she's committing me?"

"Yes," the staff member answered.

"Oh no. I don't ever want her to feel like she did this to me." And she took the pen from my hand and signed the papers herself.

Alone at 15

After I dropped my mom off at the Pavilion, I didn't go straight home. I couldn't. I was only 15, and I had just signed my mother into a mental hospital. My brain needed a minute to catch up with what had just happened. So I drove to the one place that had always felt steady—my best friend Brenda's house.

Her mom answered the door before I even knocked, like she knew I was coming. She didn't hesitate when she heard what happened.

"You're staying here," she said. No questions, no conditions. Just certainty. And for a moment, I thought maybe I would. Maybe I'd let someone take care of me for a change. But the truth was, I wasn't used to being taken care of. I'd been living as my mother's backup plan for years. I told Brenda's mom thank you, but no. I told her I was staying at my grandmother's house; she knew my stepmonster since they worked together, so she knew I definitely wasn't staying at my dad's house. She let me go but made me promise to come for supper and check in often.

From there, I went somewhere I'd never gone alone in my own car before—my dad's house. Either someone had dropped me off or my dad had picked me up and brought me there. I walked up to the front door like a guest and rang the bell.

Stepmonster answered the door. "What are you doing here?"

"I need to talk to my dad," I said.

Without breaking eye contact, she called into the other room, "Mickey, Shelly's here."

"Well, send her in!" he answered.

She did, and I walked into the other room. I found him sitting in his recliner, newspaper in hand, the TV humming in the background.

"What's going on, kiddo?" he asked.

I said, "I just had to put Mom in the Pavilion."

He lowered his newspaper and said, "Well, that's probably the best place for her."

"No, I don't think you understand. I had to take her. I had to check her in." I put emphasis on the "I" part of my statements.

He said nothing, and I started to cry.

"I don't know what you want me to do," he finally said, shifting in his seat uncomfortably.

"A hug would be nice," I said. He came over and gave me one, but it felt like a wet fish hug. I'm pretty sure Stepmonster was listening from the other room. Any sign of sympathy for me would be taken as sympathy for my mom, which she did not allow. After a few minutes, I got up and left. That was the only conversation I had with my dad during the entire time Mom was at the Pavilion.

I didn't go to stay at Brenda's. I didn't stay with my grandmother. I went home and locked the door behind me. And just like that, I was alone.

It might sound strange, but that didn't feel like that big of a shift to me. I was already used to running things on my own. I paid the bills. I got myself to school. I cooked my meals. I took care of business. My mom had been physically present but emotionally absent for a long time. She just wasn't there—not really. So when she left, the house didn't feel any emptier than it already was.

My grandmother and Brenda's mom made me come over a couple of times a week so they could feed and check on me. And Brenda came with me sometimes to visit my mom at the Pavilion. I'll never forget her face the first time we walked into that place. She clutched that visitor pass like it was her last lifeline. "Don't lose this," the staff told us. "It's your only way out." I had to tell her later that they weren't serious—they'd have let her out anyway. She may have been scared, but I wasn't. I was just there to make sure Mom was okay.

I don't remember feeling much of anything while Mom was at the Pavilion. I wasn't scared. I wasn't sad. I wasn't even overwhelmed. I just did what needed to be done. I went to school. I went to work. I visited Mom. I showed up for dinner at my grandmother's. I kept the lights on and stayed out of trouble. I was a little soldier marching forward no matter what.

That's the thing about growing up with long-term chaos. You don't fall apart when everything breaks. You go numb and compartmentalize the different parts of your life so that you can keep moving. Dissociation—when your mind checks out so your body can keep going—becomes second nature. I didn't have a word for it then, but I was already fluent in that specific language of survival.

And that, more than the hospital, more than the psychotic break of my mother, more than being 15 and alone, is what finally caused me to realize that no one was coming to save me. There was no safety net. No one was crawling out of the woodwork to make sure I was okay. It was just me. Just me, the bills, the dishes, and the silence.

And somehow, I was fine because I had to be.

Before and After

Mom's stay at the Pavilion lasted seven weeks. During that time, she had a complete and total break from reality. The kind where you take off all your clothes because you think it makes you invisible, and no one will be able to see you illegally smoking in the ward. The kind where you forget your own life. When she came out, she told me everything. When she now thought about her life before the Pavilion, it felt like reading someone else's story or watching a movie of someone else's life.

To me, it seemed like she'd pressed reset on her life, but not in a light, "New Year, New Me" kind of way. It was like she'd left one version of herself in that hospital and walked out as someone else entirely.

She even legally changed her name. Just like that, Teena Grimm became Tina Navarra. She had a new name to go with her new diet, her new habits, and her completely restructured identity. I think that was her way of surviving everything that had happened. Letting go of the weight she couldn't carry anymore by pretending it wasn't even hers.

I didn't argue with her. After what we'd been through, I figured if a new name gave her a little more peace, she could have it.

And in fairness, she did seem better—physically, at least. She quit smoking for a while and started eating healthily. She couldn't go back on prednisone; they told her that her only other option to survive was to change her diet, so she did. She got serious about nutrition, which was a huge pivot for someone who used to think a cheese sandwich with a glass of iced tea was a proper lunch. The owner of the health food store she frequented agreed to purchase a commercial-grade juicer for her and let her pay him back in installments.

Mentally, she was never what I'd call "well," but she was *clearer*. More predictable. Less fire and brimstone, more carrots and celery. And if it took obsessing over diet to keep her stable, I wasn't going to complain. Her focus had just shifted from managing her illness through medication to managing it through food.

Before, she was unstable, erratic, and physically falling apart. Afterward, she was controlled, hyper-focused, and trying—really trying—to do things differently. I think the break, as terrifying as it was, forced her to confront a possibility she hadn't let herself consider: *I might be here on this Earth longer than I thought.*

She'd lived like someone who was dying for years. She lived like she wanted, said what she wanted, and did what she wanted—consequences be damned. But after the Pavilion, there was a shift. It was like she realized, *Wait a minute. If I'm not dying yet, I'd better figure out how to live.* Part of that meant trying to stay out of the hospital; hence the health food and juicing.

For me, it meant adjusting to a new version of the same mother. She was still unpredictable, still self-focused, but now she had a cause. She no longer saw her past as part of her story, and she was ready to make up for lost time when it came to being the mother she felt I needed.

Except I'd been mothering myself—and her—for years. I wasn't going to take her stepping in at that point and trying to be Super Mom very well, but that's a story for the next chapter.

Doing Things Differently

Sometimes it takes something earth-shattering—a total collapse—to bring about real change. That's what the psychotic break was for my mom. A hard stop. A reckoning. And as much as it gutted both of us at the time, it also opened a door.

She came out of that hospital changed. She wasn't cured or healed, but she *was* different. It gave her a new lens on her health, on her choices, and on her future. She started acting like someone who might actually live long enough to regret a few things—and maybe even long enough to fix those regrets.

She embraced nutrition like it was a religion. She believed that if she followed the rules—juicing, supplements, the right foods, no smoking, low stress—she could avoid ever going back to that place again. And for a while, it worked. She went into remission for eight years. Eight years without a hospital stay, without another resection, without falling completely apart. It was the longest stretch of stability I'd ever seen from her.

Was it perfect? No, of course not. She was still my mom, still all about Tina, just with a new obsession (and a different spelling of her name). Her control issues didn't go away—they just moved from chaos to kale. But I'll give her this: She made a real effort. The Pavilion scared her straight, at least in some ways. It gave her a new mission, and in its own twisted way, it gave us both a tiny bit of breathing room.

But here's the thing I want people to understand. Drastic change might be necessary, but it can't come at the expense of the people still picking up the pieces. I was 15. I was legally emancipated and running a household completely on my own. That part didn't magically reset just because my mom started juicing carrots.

So yes, things got better for her. And yes, she did some things differently. But no, the burden didn't go away for me. It just shifted. And that's what I want readers to see clearly: When someone is sick for a long time, it's not just their story. It's the story of everyone around them. And sometimes, the person getting better won't really benefit the person who needs the most help.

If you're reading this and you're in the spot where nobody's crawling out of the woodwork to make sure you're okay, if there's no safety net, then hear me when I say this: You're not overreacting. You're not broken. And you're not alone.

In some ways, I was lucky. I had a house that was paid for. I had a dad who, even if he wasn't emotionally available, kept sending the child support check. That didn't make what I went through easy—but it did make it *possible*. Without that? I probably would've done what a lot of kids in my situation do—run away and end up on the streets.

That's one reason why I tell people about Covenant House. It's the largest private shelter program in the country for homeless teens. I worked with them for years in New Orleans. This shelter doesn't just provide a bed and a meal. They help you finish your diploma. They connect you with a job. They give you a plan. But more than that, they give you hope. And they don't just let you in and forget you—they *expect* you to make it. Because they believe you can.

And I believe that too. If you're under 18 and on the street or heading that way, look them up. Call them. Walk in the door. I know it's scary. But it's not as scary as trying to survive alone.

And if your situation isn't that severe—if you're still at home, or barely hanging on, or stuck in a house full of instability—then let this be the nudge to find someone to talk to. A counselor. A therapist. A group. There's so much available online now, and I'm telling you: *You need it.* Because of the emotional and psychological fallout of this kind of life, it doesn't always show. I didn't go to school with bruises or dirt under my nails. I bathed. I smiled. I looked fine. But I wasn't fine. I was just surviving.

That's the hardest kind of neglect for people to see because it doesn't leave marks.

So, if this chapter hit close to home and you saw yourself in these pages, don't wait for someone to come check on you. You deserve support. You deserve safety. And you deserve a future that's bigger than mere survival. There's help. Go find it.

I promise you that stepping around the trash is not the only way forward. You can look at the trash and get help that will enable you to do something about it.

Chapter 8

Emancipation Day

When Mom got out of the Pavilion after seven weeks, she acted like somebody had hit the reset button on her life. She came home full of new plans, new rules, and a whole new attitude. She was going to eat right, exercise, live differently—and parent me properly this time around.

The problem with that last one was that she was about ten years too late.

I had been on my own for a long time by then—paying the bills, taking care of my meals, and getting myself to school. I'd been fully running the household for almost two years already. Now my mother was back and ready to take the reins and be the mom, including curfews, check ins, and house rules. Don't get me wrong. I wasn't mad at her. I knew she thought she was doing what a mother was supposed to do, but there's a point of no return when it comes to parenting a kid, and I had passed that point a long time before her new plan came into play.

I couldn't unlearn the independence I'd spent years developing, but Mom didn't understand. She saw her time at the Pavilion as a big, whole-life transformation. I'm sure it was—for her. But for me, it was just another chapter of the same old story of me figuring out how to survive while the adults around me tried to rewrite the past.

What Mom didn't realize—or maybe she just didn't want to admit it—was that by the time she left the Pavilion, I had already built my own life. I wasn't looking for her to come save me. I had learned the hard way that if you wait for someone to swoop in and make life feel all better, you might be waiting forever. And I was finished waiting, thank you very much.

So when she came at me with a fresh rulebook, I did what many teenagers do.

I said, "No."

And I really meant it because I had already been surviving without her.

Legal Emancipation

Saying no wasn't new for me. I'd been saying no—with my actions, if not my words—for a long time. The reason I could stand there and look my mom dead in the eyes and tell her no was that she actually didn't have any authority over me anymore. I was already legally emancipated. Yes, at age 13, I "divorced" my parents...but not because I was trying to be some kind of teenage rebel. There was no courtroom drama. No legal battle. It was way less exciting than that. I just wanted to sign my school paperwork.

Before I had my hardship driver's license, if Mom was too sick to get out of bed, my dad would have to pick me up and drive me to school. He was always running late, and I'd need a signed note from a parent to avoid an unexcused absence.

Even after I could drive myself, I missed a lot of school running my mom back and forth to doctors' offices and the hospital. And guess what—you had to bring in a note to excuse those absences too. Plus, there were the field trip permission forms, fundraiser permission forms—you name it. I could never find anybody to sign anything.

I'd show up at school empty-handed, trying to explain why I didn't have a signature—again—and get nothing but the side-eye from the school secretary. Then she'd have to call my dad to verify where I was. It was a lot of running around for everyone involved. One day, Dad finally got tired of it. He looked at me and said, "Why don't you call Sturdevant and see what he can do so you can sign your notes?"

Wayne Sturdevant was my dad's longtime attorney—one of those good ol' boys who always knew how to get something done. So, 13-year-old me called him from the rotary phone at home and explained the situation, ending with, "So, how can I make it so I can just sign my own notes for school?"

He laughed. "Well, it's easier said than done. The only way to do that is to get emancipated."

"What does that mean?" I had no idea what getting emancipated was, but if it meant I didn't have to rely on anybody else to sign a piece of paper for me, I was in.

"Well, your parents basically just have to give you the authority to manage your own life," he replied.

I called Dad back and told him what Wayne had said.

"Isn't that pretty much what's already happening?" he asked.

"Well, yeah," I answered.

"Is *she* involved at all?" he asked. He always called Mom "she," as if she didn't have a name.

"Well, she thinks she is," I said. "But she's sick. That means she's never involved with anything."

"Okay then," he said. "Let's do it."

Only one parent needed to sign the paperwork, and Dad didn't hesitate. He signed and filed it with the court, and just like that—I was legally responsible for myself at 13 years old.

Mom didn't seem to grasp what had happened. I think she thought it was just another one of those "get through the day" Band-Aid solutions we were always throwing on bigger problems. She didn't realize it would come back around in a big way until she learned I had the authority to sign the commitment papers for her stay at the Pavilion. She also didn't know that when she came home from the Pavilion and tried to be Mom again, she wouldn't have a legal leg to stand on.

I am sure the town gossips had a field day with all of this. In a place like Amarillo, people love to have opinions about things they don't understand. They thought I had too much freedom, and they were clutching their pearls over how I was allowed to "run wild." It was funny how they sure had a lot to say about the fact that I could write my own school notes, but none of them cared enough to ask me how I was doing, drop off groceries, or sit in the ER with my mom when things went south.

At the time, emancipation didn't feel like a big, life-changing moment. It was practical and necessary—just another thing

I had to do to survive. Looking back, though, emancipation changed everything. Ultimately, it allowed me to take the steering wheel of my own life, and when Mom tried to grab the keys to the car back after the Pavilion, it was too little, too late.

I'd already found a coping mechanism to help me get through the challenges I faced.

My Coping Mechanism

By the end of the summer of my ninth-grade year, I had found something that helped me survive the day-to-day when everything around me felt like it was caving in: weed.

I didn't smoke pot to get wasted. I wasn't trying to be a rebel or cry out for attention. Honestly, it wasn't even about having fun. The only reason I smoked weed was to take the edge off so I could get through the day.

When I think back now, it's honestly a miracle I didn't slide into anything heavier. I had plenty of opportunities to try harder drugs, but I wasn't looking to obliterate myself. I just needed a little bit of quiet inside my own head, and marijuana gave me that.

Pot helped me manage the loneliness, the fear, and the never-ending pressure of trying to keep the wheels on a life I was way too young to be responsible for. It didn't make the bad stuff go away—but for a few hours, it made me feel like it was easier to breathe.

You're probably thinking weed wasn't a good idea. "It's a gateway drug." "It's not healthy to numb yourself." You know what? You're not wrong, and I don't condone it. But I know that in this season of my life, having a little numbness was one of the only reasons I made it through.

I'd been thinking about ending my life since I was 12. I didn't have a big, dramatic plan to do it; I just didn't want to deal with my life anymore. The back-and-forth to and from the hospital mixed with my feelings of being alone and alienated from my friends, plus knowing there wasn't anyone coming to save me, was heavy—it was too much. Much too much.

Smoking weed wasn't about rebellion for me. It was about getting through the day. If lighting up with a handful of friends made things doable for another day, then by God, I was going to do it. I needed a lifeline, and weed was it. I know that's not after-school special material, but nothing about my life ever was.

Supermom to the "Rescue"

Like I mentioned earlier, after Mom got out of the Pavilion, she decided she was suddenly going to be Supermom. She'd had a revelation of what a remarkable individual she was at the Pavilion, and she was ready to take on the world. I'm not sure who she thought she was, but to me, her response was almost comical. For the past seven weeks, I'd been on this planet with both feet firmly planted on the ground while she'd taken a trip in her mind. She was getting naked in her hospital room, thinking that would keep people from seeing her if she smoked, and I was going about life as usual.

Yet suddenly, she was determined that I was going to live like a "normal" 15-year-old girl.

One morning, she walked into the room and dropped a bomb.

"We need to talk about some rules around here," she said. She proceeded to lecture me about curfews and house rules. The problem was that I wasn't a typical 15-year-old girl, and I wasn't about to pretend to be one just to make her feel better. I'd been the adult in that house for years while she was sick. I had made sure the lights stayed on, the water bill got paid, and I used whatever was left over for groceries. She didn't get to swoop back in now and start barking orders like none of that ever happened.

"No, no, no," I replied. "That's not what we're going to do. I've been functioning on my own quite well, and I will continue to do so."

At first, I tried to be patient. I really did. I let my mother have her little speeches about "responsibility" and "respect," but inside, I was boiling. It wasn't just that I didn't want to follow her rules. It was that she hadn't earned the right to make them. That's when the arguments started.

She'd ask me where I was going, what time I'd be home, and who I was hanging out with. I didn't understand her then, but I do now. She wanted to believe I was still a little girl who needed tucking in and permission slips signed, but that little girl was gone. She had been for a long time, and I wasn't about to give up the hard-won independence that had kept me alive just because my mother suddenly decided she wanted to play house.

And she was *not* thrilled about my coping mechanism.

There was no "Shelly gets caught" moment. That's what most people assume when they hear this part of the story—that my mom found a joint in my backpack or smelled something funny on my clothes and met me in the living room for a sit-down intervention.

Nope. I wasn't trying to hide it. When she asked me if I was smoking weed, I told her.

"Shelly, where have you been?" she asked as I walked through the house to my room. "Have you been smoking weed?"

"Yeah, I smoke weed."

Honesty is just how I operate, then and now. If you ask me a question, you're going to get the truth—even if it's not the answer you want. And the answer I gave was *not* the answer Mom wanted.

"Why would you tell me that?" she wailed. "Why wouldn't you just lie to me?!"

"Why *would* I? You didn't raise me to be a liar!" I said.

"I wish I had not taught you so well," she said.

I laughed. "What are you talking about?"

"I wanted you to be able to build an argument, rationalize it, and deliver it to win," she said. "But I didn't want you to do it against me!"

Mom didn't want the reality. She wanted me to tell her what she wanted to hear, but I wasn't about to start lying just to make her feel better. Honesty was pretty much the only thing I had left.

Yelling at me didn't change anything, so her next move was to haul me off to Dr. Quintanella—the town's one and only psychiatrist. I don't blame Mom for taking me. What she'd been through with my sister during my sister's drug-addicted years was horrible. She didn't want to live through that nightmare again, so we went.

Now, Dr. Quintanella wasn't some slick, big-city psychiatrist. He was an old-school, tell-it-like-it-is guy who had already seen my sister during her years of actual drug addiction. If anybody knew the difference between a kid who was spiraling (my sister) and a kid who was doing her best to cope (me), it was him. So I sat in his office and answered every single question he threw at me.

"So, Shelly, what's going on in your life right now?" he asked. "Are you smoking weed?"

"Yes."

"Are you doing anything else?"

"No."

"Are you planning to start doing harder stuff?"

"No."

"How often do you smoke weed?"

"In the morning before school, and when I get home after school."

"Where?"

"It depends on who has it."

"And you're showing up at school and taking care of yourself?"

"Yes, and I pay the bills and manage the household."

"Okay. Are you sexually active?"

"No."

I laid it all out there, plain and simple. I answered every question Dr. Quintanella asked honestly, no dramatics or tears, just straight facts.

Dr. Quintanella listened and nodded along, tapping his pen on his clipboard from time to time. Then he looked at me and said, "Okay, well, you're going to be fine, but if you ever start feeling like you want to use harder stuff, come see me first."

That sounded good to me, so I agreed. We walked out of his office and met my mom in the lobby. She stood up when she saw us, ready for the bad news.

"She's fine," he said.

Mom blinked like she hadn't heard him correctly. "She's smoking pot!" she said, her voice rising.

"Yes," he answered. "And from what I can see, that's the least of her problems. She's honest, she's functional, and she's surviving in a situation where most kids would have fallen apart a long time ago. If all she's doing is smoking a little weed, you're lucky."

"Well, what am I supposed to do?" she asked.

"If it gets worse, bring her back."

"You don't want to set up anything regular with her?"

"No, I don't," he said. "If something changes, bring Shelly back. But for now, leave her alone. It's a miracle she's not a drug addict or living on the street somewhere. She's going to school. She's going to work. She's running a household. So she's a little high when she's doing it—that's her coping mechanism."

That was it. The big intervention my mom had imagined turned out to be a stamp of approval on the only coping mechanism that was keeping me sane.

The ride home was silent. Mom gripped the steering wheel like she could squeeze the disappointment out of it. I stared out the window, feeling a strange mix of relief and sadness.

It felt good to have one adult in my life tell me I was going to be fine. I was just doing what I had to do to survive, and sometimes, survival doesn't look pretty. And you know what? I was okay. The day I left Denton and started my new life in New Orleans, I never touched weed again. I didn't need to once I'd made it out.

Things didn't get easier at home after my visit to Dr. Quintanella, though. The final straw came during another one of our endless arguments about rules. After another shouting match where neither of us was willing to back down, I finally said it.

"Maybe I should just move out!"

She froze for half a second, and then, in a cold, clipped tone, she said, "Well, you can just go talk to your daddy about that."

She probably said it because she didn't think there was any way he'd agree. Her line in the sand was drawn. But what she didn't realize was that if it was her way or the highway, I'd been on the highway ever since I'd walked myself home from school at seven years old. There was no going back now.

Moving Out

After that argument with my mom, I picked up the phone and called my dad.

"Hey," I said, calm as ever. "I need to talk to you."

"Okay, Shotgun," he said. "What's going on?"

"You won't believe what this trippy woman wants to do now!"

"What?" he asked, immediately understanding who the trippy woman was.

"She's trying to be my mom," I huffed.

"Well, don't you think it's a little bit late for that?"

"Yeah! She's trying to give me all these ground rules and curfews."

"Well, you *do* need to be home, you know."

"I *am* home, Dad," I answered. "It's just that all of a sudden now she's like, 'Check in with me. Be home at this time.' She was in the hospital for seven weeks. She didn't have a clue where I was during that time. I could have been turning tricks or strung out on Amarillo Boulevard, and she never would have known it. Now all of a sudden she's concerned?" I took a deep breath. "Look, I realize she's had some kind of supermom epiphany, but would you be okay if I moved out?"

The other end of the line was silent for a moment as he thought over my question.

"Well, yeah," he agreed. "Go find something and let me know how much it costs. Try to keep it reasonable."

Dad knew I wasn't bluffing. He recognized that I'd already been on my own in every way but my physical address for a long time. I found a little fully furnished apartment with all utilities included for $165 a month. It wasn't anything fancy, but it worked, and the child support check would cover it. My dad co-signed the lease with me, and that was that.

I had my own place at age 15. I don't remember crying or celebrating. I just unpacked my things and made my bed in the one-bedroom unit that was now my home. I had a fridge, a stove, and a small table where I could eat my meals and do my homework. No one was yelling at me. There were no curfews. There was no tension. I no longer had to contend with rules that didn't make sense.

I felt free. But freedom, I quickly learned, comes with its own kind of weight. When you're 15 and living alone, nobody checks in on you. Nobody asks if you got home safe or notices if you're gone too long. You're just...on your own. But I kept going to school and making sure there was food in the fridge.

I was doing it, and every day that I woke up in that little apartment was proof that I didn't need anyone to save me. I was saving myself, even if I shouldn't have had to.

Doing Things Differently

Looking back now, it's easy to see what went wrong. My mom and I—our roles got reversed. Somewhere along the way, I stopped being the kid and started being the one who held everything together. I wasn't the one getting tucked in at night—I was the one locking the doors, checking the oven, and making sure the lights were turned off to save money on the bill.

And once that shift happens—once a kid has to become their own safety net—you can't just flip a switch and expect them to crawl back into the child role because it's convenient for you. My mom didn't understand that. When she came home from the Pavilion, she thought she could slap down a list of rules and expect me to fall in line like none of what we had been through together had ever happened.

The years she spent battling steroid psychosis had turned me into someone who *had* to be my own parent, and she couldn't just dictate her way back into a mother-child relationship with me.

As a result of all this, I eventually realized some important things that would serve me well. You can't force trust. You can't demand obedience from someone you left standing alone in the middle of a battlefield when you should have been there to fight for them and with them. If you want to rebuild something broken, you have to be willing to collaborate.

You have to sit down, eye to eye, and say, "I know I let you down. Let's figure this out together."

Mom didn't—or maybe couldn't—do that.

Mom didn't know that when she gave me the book *Games People Play*, it would come in handy when it came to managing my relationship with her too. We were stuck in what was called the Parent-Adult-Child dynamic. She was trying to parent me from a top-down position, but I wasn't a child anymore. I was an adult in every way that mattered. And adults don't respond well to being treated like children—especially when they've already been carrying the weight of two lives on their shoulders.

It's not that I didn't want a relationship with my mom. I did. But if there was going to be any hope of that happening, it was never going to come from her laying down the law. It was only ever going to come from her sitting across from me, eye to eye, heart to heart, and saying, "I see you. I'm sorry. Let's build something new."

If you have a chronic illness, don't be blind to the weight and pressure that your health issues can place on your children. Keep communicating, and do it with the help of a counselor or therapist. A professional has the tools to help you keep communication lines open with your kids, no matter how tricky the circumstances are.

That type of conversation or support didn't happen for me, and by the time I moved into that little apartment at 15 years old, I knew better than to expect that it would.

I still drive past that little apartment sometimes and am flooded with memories of what my time was like there. In the end, I only lived there for five months. I moved back into my childhood home when my mom moved to Edmond, Oklahoma, to stay with my older sister Tanya. Little did I know I was about to start a brand new adventure with Mom—an adventure that involved the dreaded "C" word: cancer.

PART 2

Nowhere to Belong

Chapter 9

Back Home, but Not the Same

W hen I signed that lease and moved into my first apartment, I thought I was finally free. At 15, with a $165-a-month rent and a little furnished place to call my own, I felt like I had clawed my way into adulthood. For the first time in years, the only expectations placed on me were the ones I set for myself. And that felt like peace.

I made my own meals. I paid my own bills. I even had a job at the health club selling memberships. I wasn't clocking in at some teen-managed fast-food joint—I was doing actual sales. I was convincing grown adults to invest in their futures with nothing but my words and a clipboard. It was a *real* job—at least, that's what I thought.

Turns out, not everybody agreed. But I'll get to that in a minute.

After a few months of settling into the quiet of my little apartment life, something happened that shook me. One day, I came home and immediately knew someone had been inside. Nothing was taken—no broken glass, no drawers rifled through—but the window near the bottom of the unit had been jimmied open just enough to let someone in. I lived alone, but I wasn't stupid. Someone I knew—or worse, someone I didn't—had broken in. They were probably just looking for a place to crash or a snack to steal. Still, it rattled me.

Not long after, the phone rang. It was Mom.

She said she had an exciting opportunity in Edmond, Oklahoma—a job at a law firm as a legal secretary. There wasn't much work for her in Amarillo, and since we'd lived in Oklahoma City before, it made sense. She said she was going to stay with Tanya, my older sister, while she got settled. It seemed like she had thought her plan through.

"Do you want to move back into the house while I'm gone?" she asked.

"Sure," I said, relieved to have a reason to leave the apartment.

I didn't think twice, and I didn't ask too many questions. I packed up my clothes, my coffee mugs, my discount pots and pans, and my bedsheets, and called my dad.

"I'm leaving the apartment," I told him.

"What are you going to do about your lease?" he asked. "You'll lose your deposit."

"Well, honestly, Dad, someone got in here the other day," I answered. "I don't feel safe anymore."

"Why didn't you tell me about it then?" I could tell he was shocked.

"Would it really have made any difference?" I asked. What was done was done. Telling him about it wouldn't have stopped it from having already happened.

"Well, I guess not," he admitted. "But I want you to be safe. I guess I should have gotten you a place on the second floor."

In the end, I did lose my $250 deposit, but it was worth losing the money to get back my peace of mind. I loaded up my things, said goodbye to my first little apartment, and moved back into my childhood home. Only this time, it wasn't me and Mom. It was just me.

What I Didn't Know

I didn't find out the truth about why my mother moved to Oklahoma City until much later. Although she did work as a legal secretary while she was there, the job wasn't the reason she went. Mom had found out she had cancer. Not the kind you talk about easily. The kind no one wants to say out loud.

It started with a fistula—a common challenge for patients with Crohn's disease. A fistula can develop when chronic inflammation causes the intestinal wall to wear away, allowing an opening to form between the intestine and the skin. She had several fistulas over the years, but this one was especially severe because it was located in the perineum, the skin between her vaginal and anal openings.

When she went to her doctor for treatment, they discovered a genital wart caused by human papillomavirus, which had caused the infection that contributed to the formation of the fistula. The doctor biopsied the tissue, and the results came back malignant. My mother had skin cancer in a place so private, so tender, and so complicated that it couldn't be treated easily. It couldn't be treated in Amarillo at all because there was no one there who specialized in that kind of surgery.

So off to Oklahoma City she went to have the skin cancer removed. Thankfully, my older sister lived there, so she wasn't alone. In my mom's case, surgery wasn't a one-and-done deal. Because of her fistula, they had to remove her skin cancer bit by bit over three consecutive days since it was in such a sensitive area. They would remove as much as they felt comfortable with for that day, send the biopsy off to see if they'd reached the margins, and then have her come back if they hadn't. On the third biopsy, they were told they had gotten to the margins. It was long, drawn out, and brutal.

She never told me about the whole ordeal. When she'd call to chat, she pretended everything was fine. No one breathed a word about cancer in my direction. Not one word. I don't know if she kept it from me to protect me or to protect herself. Probably both.

It hurt when I found out months later. Hadn't I proved I was strong enough to handle anything? And in a way, it made me question everything. If she could hide something that big…what else had I missed? I wasn't the only one missing something, though. While Mom was in Oklahoma City, dealing with her cancer, I was at home dealing with troubles of my own.

Life Alone in the Family Home

So there I was—back in the house I'd spent most of my childhood in. Only this time, it was just me.

I was 16 now, still in high school, and between my income from my part-time job and the monthly child support check from my dad, I was making it work. I was taking a distributive education class that allowed me to attend school half the day and work half the day. It sounded like a win-win. I could bring in a paycheck while still getting my high school diploma.

During the first nine weeks of the class, I was working at a health club selling memberships. I took that job seriously, and I was good at it. Thanks to my mother and Dr. Maxwell Maltz— not to mention my outgoing personality, of course—I knew how to talk to people, how to listen, and how to sell them on a better version of themselves. I believed in what I was doing, and I was doing it well. And for nine whole weeks, I thought I was doing everything right. I thought I was doing exactly what that distributive education class was designed for: learning on the job while keeping up with my credits.

So you can imagine my confusion when I got my report card and saw nothing but zeros for the class. Not just a low grade. Straight zeros for the entire nine weeks—no warning.

I marched into my teacher's office, angry and confused. "Why did I get all zeros?" I asked.

"The focus of this class is that you have a job selling something," he said. "You didn't."

"What do you mean?" I asked. Were we even having the same conversation? "I sell gym memberships to people every day!"

"That's not a real sales job."

Excuse me? I thought. I was using every tool in my toolbox to sell people on the *idea* of transformation, but in his eyes, because they weren't walking away with a physical object like a T-shirt or pair of shoes, it didn't count.

When I asked him if there was any way to reverse the zeros—and believe me, I gave him a good argument as to why he should—what he gave me was a flat-out no. To this day, I'm still not sure how he could tell me selling memberships wasn't sales when, in my opinion, being able to get people to give you money for the potential result they didn't yet have was the highest form of sales skill.

"But," he added, "I won't give you zeros next time if you go find a new job."

After going toe-to-toe with him for a while, I could tell I wasn't going to change his mind. I didn't want to fail a second quarter, so I quit my job at the health club and took a massive pay cut to get hired at Montgomery Ward, a clothing store. What else could I do?

Dating Jimmy

The one good thing about quitting my job at the health club was getting away from one of the co-owners, Jimmy. From the moment I met him, I didn't like him, even though he was my boss. I sure wasn't going to miss him. But my friend Brenda had other ideas.

"Come down to the health club with me," she begged. She'd just started dating a guy who worked there, and she didn't want to drive over to see him by herself.

"No way," I replied. "I'd just be a third wheel."

"But you wouldn't...not if you started dating someone there too. What about Jimmy? You could date him. I heard he likes you."

"Are you kidding me? That's a horrible idea. I can't stand him!"

I may not have liked Jimmy much, but I wasn't opposed to the idea of sitting in the hot tub after the health club closed. So, more often than not, when I had free time, I'd find myself joining Brenda and her boyfriend at the health club. And guess who else always "happened" to be there? Jimmy.

It wasn't long before I changed my mind about my ex-boss, and he became my new, much older boyfriend. It wasn't surprising. I'd always hung out with people older than me, and most of the boys I'd dated were older too.

I never dated anybody my own age because we didn't have a thing in common. The guys my age were still caught up in football practice and who drove what muscle car. Meanwhile, I'm sitting there thinking about getting out, paying bills, and all that would come next. They were boys, and I was already living like an adult.

Looking back, I think part of the reason I gravitated toward older people—older guys especially—was because they felt closer to the world I was already operating in. When you've already had to grow up fast, people your own age just feel like kids. And truth be told, there was something about the older ones that made me feel seen, maybe even understood. At least that's what I thought at the time. It wasn't until much later that I figured out some of them weren't trying to understand anything except what they could get *from* me instead of what they could do *for* me.

Nobody was checking on me at that point—at least no adult who *should* have been. I had taken on adult responsibilities for so long that people just stopped seeing me as a kid. I paid my bills. I showed up for work. I made it to school. That was enough to keep the questions quiet, but I was only 17. Most kids my age still had someone living in the house with them— someone they were accountable to. Someone who noticed if the lights were off or the fridge was empty. I didn't have that. I was living in a house alone, going to school, holding down a job, and no one asked, "Hey, are you okay?"

Doing Things Differently

I've thought a lot about what it means to be an unparented child. For me, being unparented started long before my teenage years. It just seemed normal. I knew that it was up to me to keep myself clothed, fed, and safe, and so I took care of things. Let me just tell you, though, when that happens, you start believing that no one will help you.

If you find yourself in a spot like I was—no parents stepping in, no one calling to check if you made it home okay, except maybe a boyfriend who's far too old for you—I want you to know that there *are* places to go, people who care, and help that doesn't come with judgment.

Had I not had a house I could go back to, I might've ended up on the street like so many others. So here's my advice: Don't wait for someone else to rescue you. If no adult is looking out for you, find one. Find a counselor. Walk into a church. Talk to a teacher. Or call an organization like Covenant House. They don't just give kids a place to sleep—they help them finish school, find part-time work, and rebuild their lives with dignity. I think so highly of what they do because, truthfully, I could've been one of those kids who ended up on the streets. And now, I want to be the one who tells you that you weren't meant to survive this alone.

On the other hand, if you're on the outside looking in—if there's a kid in your life quietly drowning under too much responsibility—be the one who steps in. You could change everything for them. You could save their life.

I had to learn how to save myself, so that's exactly what I did. I experienced some really hard circumstances during this time in my life, and one of the most difficult was just around the corner. Being responsible doesn't always mean being seen, and sometimes the hardest work goes unnoticed. I was about to find this out, and as a result, I was going to have to take drastic action to advocate for myself.

Chapter 10

Withdrawing From School

T he first time I ever talked to my high school guidance counselor was in the last quarter of my junior year. Out of the blue, I was called into the office when I arrived for class one morning.

"Hi, Shelly," she greeted me as I walked through the door of her office. She folded her hands neatly on her desk, as if she were just going to dispense some friendly chit chat instead of completely upending my future. "Sit down. We need to figure some things out."

"Okay," I said, not really sure what I was walking into.

"You're not going to have enough credits to graduate next year, so we need to talk about what you're going to have to do to make those up," she said.

This was news to me.

"Okay...," I repeated, uncertain about what she was getting at. "What do you mean I don't have enough credits?"

"Because you didn't get any credits for distributive education when you got those zeros, your overall credit acquisition was affected," she answered.

Oh yeah. That. I thought I'd done what I could to rectify that, but before I could get a word in edgewise, she carried on.

"You don't have enough base credits to graduate. You will need to come in for zero hour next year, which starts at 7:30 a.m. Then this summer and next summer—before and after your senior year—you'll need to take summer school. If all that goes well, you'll probably only need to take a couple more classes in the first semester after your senior year."

I just stared at her for a moment, stunned.

"Do you not see how difficult it's been for me to attend school because of my mother being sick?" I asked.

"Well, yes," she said, nodding.

"Okay, well, my mother's not even in the house anymore. It's just me, and I'm taking care of myself on my own. I have to work so I can pay the bills and eat. If I add even *more* school than I'm already doing, I don't think I can pull all this off."

She blinked. "Well, you don't really have much choice."

And that was the moment I snapped back because she was dead wrong.

"No," I said emphatically. "I *do* have choices."

She gave me a tight little smile, as if I didn't know what I was talking about. "Oh? And what would that be?"

"I could withdraw," I said levelly, holding her gaze.

She paused, then said, "Well, we'd have to call your parents for that."

"No, you don't," I told her. "I'm legally emancipated. Go look in your file. The papers are all there."

She raised an eyebrow. "What?"

"If you look at the attendance records, you'll see that every time someone's called the school to excuse an absence or to say I'd be late, it was me. Not a parent. Just me. Go check."

She did. She got up and walked out of the office. A few minutes later, she came back with a stack of papers in her hands and laid them in front of me.

"You're correct," she said. "Here are the withdrawal papers."

I signed them all right then and there, then I stood up and walked out of the office and out of the school for good.

Telling Dad

I headed for the parking lot, climbed into the driver's seat of my car, and sat there for a moment. Mom wasn't here, so there was no question about what I needed to do now. I drove straight to my dad's office.

He looked up when I walked in and asked, "Hey, what are you doing here, Shotgun? You on your way to work?"

"Yeah," I told him. "I'm getting ready to go to work."

He looked at the clock. "So did you get out of school early?"

I shrugged. "Got out of school. No need for that *early* part."

He narrowed his eyes. "What are you saying?"

"The office called me in and told me I wasn't going to have enough credits to graduate on time because of the distributive education teacher giving me all those zeros," I said. "Their plan to fix it was to have me go to school for almost another year."

"You're kidding me."

"Nope."

He paused for a second, then asked, "Okay. Well, what's your plan now?"

"I guess I'm just gonna go to college."

He raised an eyebrow. "Well, you'd better get your GED first."

He stood up, pulled a thick yellow and white phone book off the shelf, and threw it down on the desk in front of me. "There are some blue pages in between those yellow and white pages. Look in there for the AISD—Amarillo Independent School District. Call the main number and ask them what you have to do to get your GED."

I didn't waste time. I shuffled through the blue pages until I found the number for AISD. Then, with one finger on the number in the phone book, I dialed the numbers one by one until I was patched through.

A woman's voice answered, "Amarillo Independent School District. How can I help you?"

"I'd like to take the test for the GED."

"Oh, we're giving a test tomorrow morning if you'd like to come," she answered. No time like the present, I guess. I saw no reason to wait.

"What time?" I asked.

"8:30 a.m." She took down my name and information, then asked, "What grade level have you completed?"

I told her I was in the eleventh grade.

"Great! You've had enough schooling that you don't have to take the pretest. So just come on down and take it."

I agreed, then hung up. It was settled. Less than an hour after withdrawing from high school, I had a plan in place for my next steps.

Getting My GED

The next morning, I showed up to take the GED. I wasn't nervous. I guess I wasn't confident either. Honestly, I had no idea what to expect. I was just going. I didn't know what the test would be like or what questions would be on it. But the lady on the phone had said that I didn't need to take the pretest. I figured, what the hell—might as well see what happens.

When my yellow No. 2 pencil and I finished, the proctor looked at my results and told me I'd passed. I must not have acted as excited as she thought I should, so she said, "You know, only 56% of people your age pass this the first time."

"Oh. Okay. Thanks." I wasn't trying to impress anyone or get a pat on the back. It was just the next step.

I walked out of the testing room with my GED certificate in hand, drove straight back to my dad's office, and handed him the certificate.

He looked at it, nodded once, and said, "Well, good. Now what do you want to do?"

I'd known that question was coming, and I already had an answer. "I want to go to college."

He raised his eyebrows. He hadn't expected that. "Oh, okay. So you still want to be in school, huh?"

I nodded. "Well, I mean, I probably need to be in *some* kind of school."

Nobody had ever talked to me about college. Nobody had ever really talked to me about my future, period. I think my dad's plan for me was that I would stay local and keep working. This was the first conversation we'd ever had about college.

"Right. So, how about AC here in town?" AC was what everybody called Amarillo College, the local junior college.

"Oh, no," I said. AC wasn't even an option in my mind for one main reason. "I gotta get out of Amarillo," I told him.

He kind of blinked and said, "Okay... Well, how about Abilene Christian College?"

"What? No. Dad, Abilene is smaller than this place!"

"How about Clarendon Community College?"

"No," I answered quickly. Although an hour away, Clarendon was even smaller than Abilene. I thought I was going to scream!

He sat back in his chair, out of ideas. "Well, where do you want to go?"

"Dallas," I said. "Somewhere big, like Dallas."

And immediately, he stepped in to shrink my dreams down to size.

"Oh, no," he said firmly. "That's too big, and you'd be too far away. I can't help you there."

It wasn't really that he couldn't—he just wouldn't. His support only extended as far as what would keep me close to home. Anything beyond driving distance, anything too big or too far, and he wasn't going to help me pay for it.

Defeated, I went home and called my mom in Oklahoma.

I told her, "Well, I got my GED."

She said, "I knew you would."

Then I told her about my conversation with Dad and how he offered to send me to every small-town local college nearby. Everywhere except the one place I actually wanted to go.

"I don't know what to do," I said. "I've got to get out of here!"

"I know you do," she agreed. "I'll talk to him."

And she did. She called my dad, and they had a conversation. He told her the same thing he'd told me. I was barely seventeen, and a big city like Dallas wasn't a good idea for someone my age. He just didn't feel good about it and didn't think it was safe.

She agreed with him about that part—Dallas was huge, even back then—but she also agreed with me. She had lived in Amarillo long enough to know that it would be a bad idea for me to stay. I needed to get out of Amarillo. So she offered Dad the one thing she thought he'd agree to...and the one thing I didn't want.

She offered to go with me. Thankfully, my dad said no.

"I don't want to take care of you too," he told her. "And it's time that she shouldn't have to either."

That was the end of the discussion. I was back to square one without a backup plan, trying to figure it all out on my own.

Doing Things Differently

Looking back now, I don't regret withdrawing from school. I did what I had to do. No one was stepping in with a better plan. I also wasn't about to let teachers and school staff—who barely knew I existed—keep putting impossible hoops in front of me that I couldn't jump through. An English teacher even sat me down one morning and started to cry, saying, "If you'd have just come to class, you'd have gotten A's!" It was like they didn't even think I was trying—with everything I had been trying to juggle.

I *was* trying, though. Up until a few months before, I'd been taking care of a mother who couldn't even feed herself. Now that she was out of town, I was working, paying bills, and taking care of myself. Zeros in one single class had made the difference between me graduating on time or having to go another year. More school, earlier mornings, longer summers, and no support. No, thank you—I chose myself.

The sad thing is, those shouldn't have been my only options.

There were a hundred places where someone could have stepped in and made a huge difference in my life. The school counselor could've asked real questions about what was going on at home before dropping a rigid plan in my lap. The distributive education teacher could've had the decency to tell me my grades were zeros before it was too late. Someone could've noticed that I was alone in a house with no mom, no dad, and no backup—and offered something other than more pressure.

And my dad? He could've said, "Where do you want to go, and how can I help you get there?" Not, "I can't help you there!"

So here's what I want to say if you're in the position I was in.

You get to decide what comes next. Don't let someone else decide for you. If you need out, get out—but make a plan. Whether it's getting a GED or a job, or going to college, choose something that will allow you to earn something that belongs to you on the other side of that decision. Ask for help, even if you've been on your own a long time, and it feels like no one's listening. Keep asking.

And if you're watching someone go through what I did—maybe you're an educator, youth pastor, or coach—step in. Speak up. Offer options. If there's a young person in your life carrying adult responsibilities without adult support, ask how they're doing. Help them map out a path that doesn't end in burnout.

I didn't need—or want—someone to do it all for me. I just needed someone to say, "I see you. Let's figure this out together."

My next step was to figure out what kind of future I could build with nothing but a GED and determination. Because I was going to be leaving Amarillo soon, all right, just not in the way I thought I would.

Chapter 11

Meeting Officer Bloomfield

T he first time I met Kim Bloomfield, I didn't know he'd end up saving my ass more than once. I was just a mouthy eighth grader who got pulled over behind the wheel of someone else's car. He was a high school liaison officer watching it all go down from the sidelines.

Let me set the stage for you. It was the summer after eighth grade. I'd just finished the year out at Fannin Junior High after transferring there from Crockett. My new friends Lori and Tricia, ninth graders from Fannin, were driving around in a car that an older girl who was in beauty school had let us borrow. We were headed to Tricia's house, and as usual, I took a shortcut across the strip mall parking lot because it got us there faster. It was 8 a.m., and the lot was empty as a tomb.

Except, that is, for Officer David Sanchez in a late-model police cruiser who flashed his lights in our direction and pulled us over.

I get it—I'm small. Even though I'd had my hardship permit for over a year, the cop must've thought I looked too young to be behind the wheel. Or maybe the way I was speeding across the parking lot diagonally caught his attention. Either way, he was ready to play the big man.

"I'm sorry, Officer," I said in my sweetest voice. "I was just taking a shortcut."

"License, registration, and insurance, please," he said sternly. I started rummaging through my purse for my driver's license. He continued, "I pulled you over because you were speeding in the parking lot."

I stopped looking for my license long enough to automatically reply, "There's no speed limit in the parking lot."

I returned to feverishly digging in my purse for my license. Lori, who was sitting in the front seat, searched through the glove box for the insurance and registration.

"Here's the registration," she said, passing it to me. "But I couldn't find the insurance."

Officer David Sanchez—I'd caught a glance at his nametag when I made my smart remark about speed limits in parking lots—leaned down in the window and asked Lori loudly, "What was that you said?"

"I couldn't find the insurance, sir," she repeated.

Not wanting my friend to get in trouble, I rushed to explain. "This isn't our car. It's our friend Margo's. She's a beauty school teacher at Exposito Hair Design, now called the Exposito School of Hair Design. We were on our way back over there. We went to pick up breakfast for all the students at the donut shop."

Immediately, Officer Sanchez yanked open my door. "That's it! Get out! We're going downtown."

"What? Why?" I wasn't sure what was going on, but this seemed ridiculous to me. "Are you kidding me? We didn't do anything!"

"You didn't have insurance, and you were speeding in the parking lot," Officer Sanchez said.

"Oh, come on," I scoffed. I never could keep my mouth shut. "I mean, seriously? Why do you have to be such a jackass?"

"That's it, verbally assaulting an officer," he said, ready to throw the book at me. "Let's go. Right now."

While his partner went around to the other side of the car to speak with my two friends, Officer Sanchez ordered me to step out of the car.

I flatly refused. Again, he told me to step out of the car so he could cuff me.

"Are you kidding me?" I hit him with a stream of profanity. "You can't do that, you motherf–!"

"Okay, that's resisting arrest," he smirked, enjoying watching me get worked up. "And another charge for verbally assaulting an officer."

"Oh, you wanna see resisting?" I yanked my elbow out of his grasp.

"And, another one." You could almost see him mentally tallying the charges in his head. "You just won't learn, will you, girl?"

Before we knew it, we were in the back of that late-model cruiser on our way to the station, and he was stacking on the charges like they were poker chips and he was getting ready to win the pot of his life.

"Okay, that's assaulting an officer. That's two…three…four. That's another one." He kept going, and so did I. By the time we got to the station, he had 14 charges piled on, and he was sure I'd be put in jail.

If not for Officer Kim Bloomfield, who happened to be at the station that morning, I might have been put in jail because Officer Sanchez wasn't done throwing out trumped-up charges yet. I didn't know Bloomfield. He was the local high school liaison, and I wasn't even in high school yet. He hadn't been the one to arrest me, but he *was* the one who ended up making sure I didn't get swallowed by the system.

Sanchez turned us over to the officers at the station, one of whom was Officer Bloomfield, and went to fill out the paperwork—or so we thought. As we were waiting for processing, he came strolling back in, holding a burned-up joint.

"Well, look what I found, ladies," Sanchez sneered. He held up the roach like it was a key piece of evidence for a murder trial. Except there was one problem.

There was nothing in that car when we got pulled over. I knew it, my friends knew it, and Sanchez knew it too. The only way a joint could have ended up there that day was if he planted it. I was instantly mad enough to spit nails.

"You're full of shit," I said, looking him dead in the eye. "That wasn't in the car. You planted it."

And that's when Bloomfield spoke up for me. From that moment, we struck up an unlikely friendship. I didn't know it then, but he'd end up being my ally more than once. He just kept showing up, even when nobody else did. Suddenly, it felt like I wasn't dealing with life all alone.

That doesn't mean we didn't get in trouble for our run-in with Sanchez, though. We didn't get charged, but Lori and Tricia were in deep water with their parents. And me? Well, I couldn't even call my mom to come get me. I was the one in the household who drove, remember? So I had to face it myself. Lori, bless her heart, ended up having to go live with her dad after that. She tells me now it was the best thing that ever happened to her. She ended up getting married to my favorite cousin and having kids, and then, years later, grandkids. She still says she wouldn't change a thing, but back then, I felt like I'd derailed her whole life.

"It's Me."

Bloomfield became a steady presence in my life after that first run-in. By then, I guess you could say we had an understanding. He wasn't just a cop. He was one of the only adults in my life who *saw* me and gave a damn whether I made it through life or not.

The second time Bloomfield stepped in and spoke up for me also came about because of a car, but this time, the car was parked. A girlfriend and I were parked behind my old elementary school one night, just sitting and talking. I was smoking weed, and she was working on a bottle of beer. We had the windows cracked about an inch to let the smoke drift out. It was chill. No big deal.

"Pass me that joint," my friend whispered.

"Okay, here," I said. I nudged her with my elbow to take the joint from my hand.

"What?" she asked, confused.

"Here's the joint," I waved it in front of her. "Take it."

"No, I don't want it," she said.

"Yeah, you do. You just asked me for it."

"No, I didn't," she denied.

Inwardly, I rolled my eyes. *Whatever.* Then I heard it again.

"Pass me that joint."

I was starting to get irritated. "Okay. Here!" I tried to hand it to her.

"What? I don't want that!" she insisted.

"Well, quit asking me for it if you don't want it, then," I replied.

"I didn't ask you for it!"

"We're the only two people in the car. Who else could it be?"

"It's me," said a deep voice from right outside my window.

I damn near jumped out of my skin.

Apparently, two cops had rolled up behind us in the alley without us noticing. One was standing at my friend's window, one at mine. Turns out, she really wasn't the one asking.

They pulled us out of the car and split us up. One officer put me in his cruiser, and the other one took her in my car. They drove us separately to the station, and the whole way there, my friend nervously tried to reason with the officer (which she relayed to me in detail later).

"Listen, my dad is a court reporter for Judge Poff. This is going to be bad news. Is there any way you can *not* do this?" she begged.

"No. No, we're doing it," the officer replied. "You know, your friend's going to sell you out. She was the one holding the weed, but you know she's gonna sell you out and say it's yours."

"No way," she said. "She wouldn't do that."

Inside, though, she was sweating bullets and praying I wouldn't. Her dad was strict. Her parents wouldn't have had a problem with her drinking, but they'd die if they thought she was smoking pot. That would have been BIG trouble for her, so she really didn't smoke weed. Meanwhile, I didn't drink, but I had the weed.

When we got to the station, it was probably one or two in the morning. They kept my friend and me separated, but I immediately told them the drugs were mine. "It was mine. She was just drinking."

Because we were Amarillo High School students, the officers called Bloomfield. He came down in the middle of the night.

He walked into the conference room they'd stuck me in, took one look at me, and asked, "What the hell are you doing here?"

"Nothing good," I answered smartly.

"Yeah, I can see that," he replied, not letting me off the hook. "Who do you want me to call—your mom or your dad?"

"Call my dad to get me out and my mom to pick me up," I said. "But first, what's going to happen to my friend?"

"We've already called her mom, and she's coming to pick her up."

"Okay, so nothing's gonna happen to her?"

"No, they think all she did was drink beer."

"Well, that's all she *did* do, you know?"

He picked up the phone and called my dad.

"Hello?" I could hear my dad's voice through the phone.

"Hello, Mickey Grimm? We've got your daughter down here at the station. They found her in her car with some marijuana behind the elementary school."

"Well, did anybody ask to search her car? Did they have a warrant?" Dad asked.

"No, sir," Bloomfield answered. "But we're letting her go."

"Well, that's a good idea, because I don't want to have to get Judge Poff out of bed right now," he said. Judge Poff's name sure got a workout that night.

That was that. Then Bloomfield called my mom, and she came and picked me up.

Once again, Bloomfield had shown up before things got too deep. Looking back now, I realize Bloomfield could see I was on the edge. He knew who I ran with and that I had enough smarts to get out. He just wasn't sure I had enough support to make getting out stick. I wasn't in and out of trouble all the time. Just often enough that if the wrong person had stepped in instead of Bloomfield, my story could've turned out very differently.

Kristi and Sami

Even after I left school and no longer had the school liaison connection with Bloomfield, he still checked in often, and I was glad. After I pulled myself out of school, things got quiet. My mom was still in Edmond. I wasn't hanging with Brenda much anymore because we'd ended up at different high schools. Instead, I became good friends with a girl named Kristi.

Kristi and I clicked fast. Trauma kids can spot each other a mile away. Her mom was a total mess, too, but mentally, not physically. Kristi's mom worked in radio, and by the time Kristi hit junior high, her mom was seriously unstable. Kristi ended up moving in with her dad and stepmom in Amarillo around eighth grade. She was the oldest, the one who had to keep it all together. Sound familiar?

Her dad and stepmom loved me. I mean, they genuinely loved me. I drove this little Volkswagen Bug that always died at stoplights. Her dad—a small engine mechanic out at Bell

Helicopter—taught us how to jump out, grab a screwdriver, and reconnect whatever it was that made it spark again. One of us would be under the hood, and the other would be in the driver's seat. We were like an efficient pit crew, she and I. She drove, I popped the clutch, and we carried on.

Years later, even after Kristi had moved to Japan, I'd drive to Dallas just to see her and her parents when she went home to visit. Her stepmom even asked to talk to me right before she passed. That's the kind of family they were. They were good people who treated me like I was one of their own.

But one day, Kristi got tangled up with this younger girl—we'll call her Sami, though I can't quite remember her actual name. Sami was rough around the edges, and I mean *rough*. She lived on the east side and was being raised by her single dad. That girl loved every basketball player in school (and I do mean *every*). She wasn't my speed. She wasn't Kristi's either, but Kristi seemed to like her. I think Kristi felt more sorry for Sami than anything. She didn't have a lot of girlfriends.

Kristi called me one night and said, "Hey, you wanna hang out? I've got some Valium. You've gotta try it."

"Okay, well, what does that do?"

"It relaxes you," she said.

The idea of relaxing sounded like a vacation to me. We met in the parking lot of my boyfriend Jimmy's apartment complex and split one.

That thing knocked me out cold. I slept like the dead, and when I finally woke up, I said to Kristi, "Don't ever give me that again. Where did you get that?"

She laughed and said, "I got it from Sami's dad."

That stopped me. "Wait—Sami's *dad* gave you prescription meds?"

"Yeah," she said, "he's cool. You should come over with me sometime. We hang out over there and get high. It's no big deal."

I wasn't so sure about getting high with Sami's *dad*, but who was I to judge? Maybe it was curiosity. Perhaps it was stupidity. I said okay, and later that week, we went.

Sami's house was a circus. There were lots of people coming and going, and the whole place was filled with noise and chaos. There was too much activity going on for this to be a regular household. It didn't take a genius to figure out what was going on—Sami's dad was dealing, and not small time.

We didn't stay long. I didn't want to. That place gave me a knot in my gut. I wasn't scared often, but at that house? Being at that house made me nervous. I didn't belong there, and I knew it. The way people moved, the way they looked at you, all the things that were *not* being said—you could feel the danger in the air like static.

I never went back there again. I probably saw Sami a time or two after that, but I didn't develop a close friendship with her. I may not have always made the smartest choices, but I *was* smart enough to know not to go back to that place.

Little did I know that my decision to stay away from that whole situation wasn't going to be enough to keep me out of trouble.

Lunch at Taco Villa

A few days after that weird night at Sami's dad's place, Officer Bloomfield called again. When I pulled myself out of school, I think he got worried about me because that meant he couldn't check on me at school anymore. He knew I was living alone, which he wasn't a fan of for a 17-year-old. My mom was gone, my dad wasn't around, and it seemed like Bloomfield just felt like *somebody* needed to keep an eye on me. He could tell I was at a fork in the road and could easily go one way or the other. I'd either go down the right path or the very, very wrong one.

Bloomfield was determined to do what he could to make sure I chose the right path.

"Hey, Shelly," he said that day. "Let's go grab lunch."

So we did.

We went to the town's favorite—Taco Villa. Taco Villa had cheap, Mexican fast food, and it was better than one of those national chains. There was one not far from the high school, but not so close you'd run into a crowd of kids. That's the one we picked.

We walked in and got in line. Right away, I noticed two guys sitting at a table—Albert and Gary. I'd gone to school with Gary since junior high, and I knew Albert from high school. I said hi like normal. We weren't close friends, but we ran in the same circles. It would have been unusual for me not to acknowledge them.

They didn't say much back, which I thought was a little odd. But like I said, it's not like we were super close or anything.

Bloomfield and I got our food and sat down at a table. We did our usual song and dance where he asked me how things were going, I told him things were fine, and he cautioned me to be careful and take care of myself. Then we went our separate ways, and I didn't think anything of it.

I mean…it was only Taco Villa. I just had lunch with a guy who happened to be a cop and cared whether or not I ended up dead or in jail. I sure didn't think that one plate of tacos was enough to put my life in danger. But apparently, someone else did.

The Party to End All Parties

I hadn't been out of school long—maybe a couple of weeks— but it wasn't unusual for my school friends to show up at my house with a keg and a story. "This got delivered to my house by accident," they'd say, grinning like they'd pulled off a magic trick. I'd roll my eyes and say, "Delivered by accident, riiiiight." But then I'd shrug and tell them, "Fine, take it to the backyard."

My friends knew that pretty much anything went at my house, so that was pretty standard for a Friday night around my place. But that spring break, things heated up several more notches. The party that happened that weekend ended up being the last party I ever had at that house.

I'm not sure how many people showed up. All I know is they rolled in with not one, not two, but three kegs, and it was like the floodgates opened. People I hadn't seen in forever came pouring in—old friends from Crockett, Bonham, and Amarillo High all came to my house. A lot of them were people I'd known since we were in grade school. They were used to seeing me with it all together. They knew the Shelly who held down a job, ran her mom around to doctor's appointments, and showed up at school sporadically.

What they walked into that night was chaos. I know for a fact there was coke being done in one room, mushrooms in another, and crank in the bathroom. It was a damn smorgasbord of drugs, booze, and bad decisions—and it was all under my roof.

This was the early '80s, back when North Texas was a hotbed for drug activity. There were high-volume drug dealers, like Sami's dad, living just miles away. And I was so naive back then. I mean, I knew half the classes from '81 to '84 were likely going to finish their educational endeavors in the pen, but it never once occurred to me that I was putting myself in danger.

After all, the kids my age who were there thought my living situation was pretty cool. What 17-year-old wouldn't think it was awesome to have a three-bedroom house to themselves with no parents looking over their shoulder? It was at that party that people started to realize I wasn't in school anymore. It clicked for a lot of them: "Wait, Shelly's not just skipping class. She's out." And with that realization came questions. Where were my parents? Why was a house full of minors doing hard drugs while I played hostess in the middle of it all?

That party made people talk, but not just in a "wow, Shelly is so cool" type of way. Because there were other characters I wasn't even aware of watching from the background. What they saw was a teenage girl living alone and hosting a blowout party, with people of all ages coming and going with drugs and dating a man almost a decade older. Yet she was also trotting around town having lunch with a cop.

It didn't take a detective to see how that might raise some red flags, but I was blind to it all. I didn't know I'd gotten on the radar of the wrong kind of people—the kind of people who were starting to think about how easy it would be to just quietly make someone like me disappear.

Doing Things Differently

Looking back, it's easy to see where the alarms should've gone off—but when you're living in it, the noise of everyday chaos can drown out even the loudest warning signs. Remember the trash falling out of the sky illustration I talked about in an earlier chapter? I was still living right in the thick of it. Independence without oversight isn't freedom. At 17, having a house to myself sounded like a dream. But dreams can turn into nightmares fast when no one is watching out for you. Just because I could run the show didn't mean I should have been left to do so.

And having people around doesn't mean you're not alone. Yes, I had people showing up every weekend with a keg, but they just wanted a place to party with no rules. And that made me a target—not just for gossip, but for real danger. That extreme kegger? That wasn't just a blowout party. That was the moment many people realized for the first time that I was alone. And it's when I ended up on the radar of people who didn't have my best interests in mind.

The truth is, when adults look the other way, kids can fall through the cracks and into places they were never meant to be. Sure, my dad always got me out of trouble, but never stepped in to keep me out of it in the first place. And he didn't make sure I didn't fall right back in. The people who should have seen the red flags and helped me didn't. Instead, I ended up catching the attention of the wrong people.

Yet through it all, there was one person who just kept showing up. Officer Bloomfield didn't owe me anything. He was the liaison officer for my entire high school, which had several hundred students, but he still kept checking in with me. That kind of consistency matters more than grand gestures. Sometimes, just being the person who notices can save a life.

Officer Bloomfield was trying to help me. He'd already gotten me out of trouble twice, but the stakes were getting higher now. I was hanging out with people who were legal adults, and even though I didn't know it yet, if I wasn't careful, I was going to end up being another statistic.

Chapter 12

Who Put a Hit Out on Me!?

A week or so after lunch at Taco Villa and the blowout party, the phone rang and woke me up. I was dead asleep in my bed with the blackout shades pulled down at 1:30 in the afternoon. I could sleep like the dead, and it was my day off. Let me tell you, whenever I had the chance to sleep in, I took it.

"Hey, Shelly, are you awake?" It was Bloomfield.

"Not really," I mumbled, squinting at the clock. "You just woke me up."

"Sorry. Look, I need you to do something for me." His tone shifted in a way that told me I'd better wake up and fast. "I need you to look out the window—but not your bedroom window. I want you to go to a different window, maybe in the next room. And don't make it obvious."

I sat up, becoming instantly alert. I could tell something was off, but I didn't ask questions. I grabbed the phone—thankfully, I had a cord long enough to stretch across the entire house—and carried it with me into my mom's bedroom. Carefully, I peeked around the edge of the curtain and saw a white car parked across the street. A man sat alone in the driver's seat.

"There's a beat-up old white car across the street," I said. "Some guy's just sitting in it."

"That car's been there all night," Bloomfield said. "I saw it on my way home yesterday, and just for the hell of it, I ran the plates. The guy's got a record with a rap sheet as long as your arm."

My throat felt like it dropped into my stomach. *What is going on?* I thought to myself as Bloomfield continued.

"This morning, I drove by again, and the car was still there. So I started asking around, trying to find out who he runs with."

Something in the way he said it told me I wasn't going to like what he had found out, and I was right.

"Shelly, someone wants to take you out. Word is out that they are willing to pay for it too."

I sat down hard on the edge of the bed. "Wait, what?" I said. "Like...like...a *hit*?"

"Yeah. Somebody wants you dead."

My mind was spinning. Maybe I was still asleep. I thought, *This had to be a nightmare or something, right?* "Why, Bloomfield? I don't get it. Why would somebody want to kill me?"

"They think you're a narc."

I laughed. The whole situation was so surreal, but I could tell he was being serious. "Who the hell do they think I'm narc-ing on?"

"You know that girl, Sami?" Bloomfield asked. He was talking about Kristi's friend. The one whose dad's house I'd been to recently—the place I couldn't wait to leave.

"Yeah, I know her. Kind of. My friend Kristi is friends with her, so we've hung out a couple of times. Why?" I wasn't sure what Sami had to do with any of this.

"Her dad's one of the biggest dealers in town," Bloomfield continued. "You were seen at his house. Then remember how you stopped and said hi to those two guys at Taco Villa when we were having lunch? Well, Albert's been dealing for Sami's dad."

It hit me like a ton of bricks. That awkward vibe from Albert and Gary at lunch the other day hadn't been my imagination. They had seen me with Bloomfield and gotten suspicious. They assumed the only reason I'd be seen with a cop was that I was feeding him information.

I wasn't, but in that world, suspicion is enough to get you killed.

"Okay," I said quietly. "What do I do?"

"I want you to pack a bag," Bloomfield said. "Stay in the house, and don't call anyone or tell anyone. I have to head back to the high school to direct traffic. If anything happens, call emergency—but I don't think it'll come to that. I'll be back after school, so be ready to leave."

I agreed, then hung up as the full weight of the situation I'd stumbled into sank in. I hadn't sold drugs. I hadn't talked to the cops. I'd gone to Sami's house once, out of curiosity, and had lunch with a guy who happened to wear a badge. That's it.

And now someone wanted me dead.

When a Cop Tells You To Run, Run

You know how you think you're grown because you've been doing grown-up things? Paying bills, cooking your own meals, holding your own little world together? Well, let me tell you, nothing reminds you just how young—and alone—you really are like finding out there's a stranger parked outside your house, waiting to kill you.

The fact that there wasn't even a parent or family member of any kind who could help me made things feel way worse. All I had was a cop telling me to pack a bag and get the hell out of Dodge.

I listened to him, though, and I didn't call anyone outside of a select few people I saw in person before I left Amarillo. The only people who would know were Kristi, Brenda, and my boyfriend Jimmy—and I don't think they even believed me when I told them why. I packed a small bag—just enough to get by for a few days—and then I sat down and waited. Thankfully, I didn't have to wait long.

As good as his word, Bloomfield came back around 4:00 p.m. He parked down the street a bit so he wouldn't draw attention, then called the precinct, who called me and patched him through.

"You ready? I'm here. Time to go," he said.

I grabbed my bag, got in my car, and backed out of the driveway. Bloomfield followed me down the street and out onto the main street in his squad car to make sure the white car didn't chase after me.

I was a little concerned about leaving Amarillo right then, as it was going to get dark soon, so I drove to Jimmy's apartment. He had just sold his stake in the health club and was getting ready to move to New Orleans, where his brother lived, so there were moving boxes everywhere. I wandered into the kitchen, where he was making barbecued chicken for Brenda, her boyfriend, and the two of us to eat later that night.

Unceremoniously, I announced, "Guess I'm not staying in Amarillo either."

He put down the chicken and looked at me like I was nuts. "What are you talking about?"

I told him everything about the car, the hit, and what Bloomfield told me to do. And like I said, I could tell he didn't believe me. At the moment, though, that was the least of my worries. I didn't need him to believe me. I just needed a place to crash for one night.

"Look, can I just stay here tonight?" I asked. "I'll leave first thing in the morning."

"Yeah, of course. But where will you go?"

"Edmond," I said. "My mom is there with my sister."

I didn't sleep much that night, but in retrospect, I don't think anyone would blame me for that. You don't sleep easily when someone out in the world has hired a killer to take you out. Especially not when the only person looking out for you is a police officer who isn't even technically responsible for you. I'm so glad Bloomfield chose to take on that responsibility, though, even for a short time in my life.

After all, Bloomfield didn't owe me anything. He could've looked the other way and let it all play out. I wasn't really his problem, and I'd caused him enough trouble as it was. But he called, warned me, and gave me a way out.

You had better believe I took it.

The Disappearance Nobody Questioned

You'd think that when a teenage girl disappears out of the blue, people might ask questions, but no one came looking for me. As far as I know, when I left Amarillo, no one called the house. No one put up missing person posters. Everyone just assumed I'd dropped off the face of the Earth. Years later, people told me they thought I'd died. That's how invisible I'd become by then. I'd been carrying the weight of a grown woman for so long that people forgot I was still a kid.

Nobody was checking on me. Not my dad nor my mother. Not any adult who should've noticed that a teenage girl was suddenly gone. Bloomfield knew I had a father. He'd talked to my dad before. Both times I got picked up, I told him to call my dad. But he didn't go to him this time. Bloomfield didn't even mention my dad in this instance.

Why? Because I think he knew it wouldn't matter. My dad might've gotten me out of whatever jam I was in when it came to smoking weed and cussing out cops, but I would've gone right back to being alone. And this time, being alone was *the problem*. Being alone could've gotten me killed. So Bloomfield called *me* and said, "Pack a bag, and don't tell anyone you're leaving."

He was doing the best he could—above and beyond, really, for someone who didn't have a family connection to me. I wasn't even 18 yet. That whole situation wasn't something a teenage girl should've had to handle by herself. But that's the thing about kids who carry adult responsibilities—people stop checking on you. They assume you're fine, because you've been pretending to be fine for so long that they've forgotten you *were* pretending.

Doing Things Differently

Looking back now, I realize just how lucky I was that Officer Bloomfield noticed a teenager on her own and cared enough to look out for her. Without him, I could have ended up face down in a ditch somewhere.

Luck isn't a good strategy, though. Actually, it's not a strategy at all.

That's the takeaway I want you to hear loud and clear, especially if you're the one carrying too much or you know someone who is.

When you're young and living alone, when the adults in your life are either checked out or too far away to see what's really going on, it's easy to fall through the cracks. And the last thing you want to happen is for those cracks to turn into graves. No kid should be in a position where a police officer—not a parent, not a guardian—is the only one stepping in to say, "It's not safe here. You need to go."

That's not how it's supposed to work.

If I'd had someone living with me—an aunt, a dad, anyone—Bloomfield wouldn't have called me. He would've come to the house and talked to the adult. That's what should've happened. But there was no adult. There was only me, and I was still a kid, no matter how grown I looked on paper.

If you're reading this thinking, "Well, you were just smoking weed. It couldn't have been *that* serious." Let me stop you right there. Remember the raging kegger just a few weeks earlier? Things were accelerating quickly. Even if you think you're just dabbling, just tagging along, just going to someone else's house for a quick visit, you never know who else is in the room. You never know whose business you're brushing up against. You never know when something small can turn dangerous really fast.

All I did was say yes to visiting a friend's house, then showed up for tacos. All I did was let my friends in when they knocked on the door on a Friday night. Yet those simple occurrences could've been the end of me.

So if you're in that world—or if someone you love is on the edge of it—know this: it's not just about *what* you're doing. It's about who else is doing it beside you and how quickly you can get dragged down with them.

I wasn't always in the right place, but I *was* smart enough not to go back when I realized I was in the wrong one. And to stay safe, to stay alive, I was about to put Amarillo in my rearview mirror—and I wouldn't return to my hometown again for more than a decade.

PART 3

Amarillo in the Rear View Mirror

Chapter 13

Goodbye, Amarillo

A t sunrise the next morning, I loaded up my VW Beetle and took Interstate 40 east out of Amarillo.

I didn't drag things out with long goodbyes or dramatic farewells. As far as most people were concerned, I just vanished. All I took was a packed bag and whatever was left of my peace of mind, which wasn't much. My brain was still trying to catch up with what had happened and figure out what in the world I was going to do next. Basically, I was internally freaking out.

Great, now what am I going to do? I'm not sure what I had in mind, but this was definitely NOT it. The LAST place I want to be is with my sister in freaking Oklahoma City. Man, I hope I have enough gas to get there!

I made it to Edmond by late that morning and drove straight to Tanya's house, where she lived with her husband and two small children. I hadn't called first, and this was before the days of cell phones, so they had no idea I was coming. I sat in the driveway for a few moments, staring at the house with dread and wondering what kind of reception I was going to get.

There was only one way to find out. Sighing, I dragged myself out of the car, walked up to the front door, and knocked.

"Surprise!" I said with a forced smile when my sister answered. She was shocked.

"Shelly! What are you doing here?"

"Well, I…" I began, but she was already yelling back into the house for my mom.

"Mom, Shelly's here!" (At that time, my sister was still calling my mom, Mom.)

They ushered me and my overnight bag inside. I was immediately swarmed by my young niece and nephew and my cocker spaniel, Beau, who had traveled to Oklahoma with Mom. Finally, everyone calmed down enough for us to talk.

"Seriously, Shelly," Mom said. "What's going on? What are you doing here?

I knew I had to give them a reason for my visit, but I wasn't ready to tell them the whole story—not even my mom.

"You know how somebody broke into my apartment a while back? My cop friend didn't think it was safe for me to stay in Amarillo right now. You know how bad it is with drugs and stuff. So…here I am."

They bought it, and I let them. What else was I supposed to say? "Hey Mom, someone's got a hit out on me because I accidentally ran into a drug dealer's runner while eating tacos with the local high school liaison officer?"

Yeah, I didn't see that going over very well. What's wild is, we were both hiding things from each other. I guess that kind of made it even. She didn't tell me she had cancer. I didn't tell her someone wanted me dead.

It wouldn't take long for us to realize that staying with my sister was not going to work. But before we tried to solve that problem, we were going to celebrate.

Where to Next?

"All right, we're going out!" Tanya declared. We weren't super close, but Tanya *was* happy to see me. She decided that she and her husband, Jeff, would ask her in-laws to watch the kids, and then the four of us would hit the town and go dancing.

On the way there, I said, "So which one of us is going to be Tanya?"

"What do you mean?" asked my sister, confused. The county we were in was a dry county at the time, so that meant the dance hall couldn't serve alcohol. You were allowed to bring your own, though, so everyone had to be 18 to enter. I was only 17. In my eyes, though, that was not a problem.

"I just use your ID," I replied nonchalantly, rummaging around and pulling an ID out of my purse.

"What are you talking about?" she asked, turning around to glare at me from the passenger seat. "What do you mean, 'I just use your ID'?"

I held it up so she could see it. "Well, technically mine says Texas and yours says Oklahoma, but it's your ID."

"Let me see that!" she demanded, swiping it out of my hand.

"Okay, geesh!" I said, holding my hands up, palms out. I leaned back and watched her as she carefully inspected it. Sure enough, it was her ID. Her birthdate. Her name. And my photo.

"How is *your* picture on my ID?"

"I stole it out of your purse and went to the DMV in Texas. I told them I'd moved and needed to change my address, and they did it. They put my address on it and retook the picture. And now I'm Tanya Grimm, age 25. Ta-da!"

Tanya was dumbfounded, but my brother-in-law Jeff snorted in amusement from the driver's seat. He thought it was hilarious, but Tanya elbowed him and then shot him a glare. You probably wouldn't get away with it today, but back then, things were a lot less strict, and we looked enough alike that they actually thought I was Tanya and had lost my license.

In the end, we decided to let me be Tanya and hope they wouldn't ask the real Tanya to see her ID. They didn't, and Jeff spent the rest of the night jokingly calling me "wife."

That is, until I met and started dancing with an older guy. Of course, it wasn't the guy's fault. He thought I was over 18. He didn't know about the two Tanyas, so how else could I be in a club like that? But my brother-in-law knew I was underage, and he had a conniption fit—quietly, of course, since he didn't want us all to get in trouble at the club. The moment we got home though, he let us know how he felt about the situation.

"You can't stay here," he declared to Mom and me. He turned to Tanya while jabbing a finger in my direction. "She can't stay here. I can NOT be responsible for her. No way!"

I wasn't surprised. I had known we wouldn't be staying. Mom had a way of wearing out her welcome, and she'd been there for months already. Plus, there were two of them and two kids in an already too small house. It just wouldn't have worked. The problem was, I didn't really have a plan for what happened next.

Neither did Mom, but that didn't stop her from confidently replying, "Well, of course we're not going to stay. Just give us a couple of days to figure out where we want to go, and then we'll be out of your hair."

Headed South to the Gulf Coast

To Mom, this would be just another grand adventure. She started throwing out ideas as if we had all the time, money, and options in the world.

"I don't want to live up here where it's cold," she said. "I want to live somewhere where it's warm."

"Mom, that's crazy," I protested. Already, we were falling back into our old patterns of her being the dreamer and me being the voice of reason. "We can't just take off and go. We don't have any money. I don't even have any of my stuff."

"Sure, we can!" When she was in one of these moods, there was no changing her mind. That was Mom—100% free-spirited energy, 0% plan or logic.

And it wasn't like I had much choice. At that point, I was kind of at the mercy of whatever harebrained scheme she came up with. I wasn't doing drugs anymore—I'd left all of that behind for good in Amarillo. That was a good thing, but it also meant there was nothing to take the edge off my feelings to help me relax. That meant my anxiety was through the roof, and I felt like I was crawling out of my skin.

It also didn't help that for the first time in my life, I was away from home and *completely* dependent on my mom. That didn't feel right to me.

So the new plan—well, *her* plan—was to head down to the Gulf Coast and stay with her sister, my Aunt Terri. I had a cousin, Cindy, who was my age, so I think in my mom's mind, we'd just magically show up, crash at Terri's, and I'd enroll in junior college there. Her plan was going to fall into place, and the how of it all was just details we could iron out later.

My mom was building sandcastles again, and as usual, she was bringing me along for the ride. To me, anything sounded better than where I'd just been. As bad as things were in Amarillo though, I knew this wasn't really a solid plan.

Too bad it was the only plan we had.

It wasn't more than a couple of days later that we'd rented a U-Haul trailer and packed up my mom's car. Off we went—me, Mom, and Beau, the cocker spaniel. We were running on fumes, hope, and whatever vision she had in her head of the Gulf Coast.

I should have realized things were going too smoothly to last. But ready or not, we were on the way there.

And guess what? They weren't ready.

Running on Fumes

We pulled out of the driveway in my mom's white sedan, waved goodbye, and headed south. We had zero *actual* plans and even less money. Plus, I was manic. I mean, *manic*—the weed was still working its way out of my system, and it was rough. I don't remember sleeping or where we stopped for the first few days. My anxiety was through the roof, and I felt like my brain was running faster than the wheels on that U-Haul trailer.

At one point, we were traveling on LA Highway 1—this was before I-49 existed—so no interstates were cutting through Louisiana the way they do now. Just little backroad highways, dark as pitch, no lights, nothing. It had to be around 10 p.m., and I looked down at the dashboard and noticed the fuel gauge was hovering on about an eighth of a tank.

"Mom," I tapped her on the shoulder. "We have less than a quarter of a tank of gas. Next gas station we see, we gotta stop."

As we reached the outskirts of what had to be the smallest town ever, we passed a sign that read "Next gas 19 miles".

"Mom, look, there's a Texaco," I pointed up ahead, where I could see the sign with the tell-tale red star with the green T in the middle. "The next one's not for another 20 miles. We need to stop here."

She took one look at the rickety gas pumps and shady characters hanging around outside the station and just kept driving.

"We're not stopping there," she stated firmly.

"But we're almost out of gas," I protested. "Better to stop here than run out of gas and have to walk out here in the boondocks in the middle of the night!"

"We're just gonna pray," she said, unconcerned. That was my mother. "We're not stopping here."

"That's a great plan, Mom," I muttered, not holding back on the sarcasm. "Thanks."

Honestly, I thought we were probably going to die out on that road. There were no lights and no other cars around. No Google Maps or GPS to guide us. We had no idea where the next gas station was. All we knew was we were somewhere past Shreveport in north Louisiana, an area full of tiny towns you now only hear named on crime shows and podcasts.

But somehow, we made it. We coasted into Alexandria, home of England Air Force Base, on fumes. Thank God, there was a BX (base exchange) station that was open 24-7. We saw lights from the base in the darkness beaming at us like a beacon of hope, and we knew we were going to be okay. When we pulled up to the pumps, we opened the car doors, got out, and kissed the ground.

Then we laughed our asses off, borderline hysterical. It was a *miracle*. Mom might have said it was God looking out for us because we were destined for greatness. But no, this was just

God protecting two idiots. I swear, He was like, "I've got plans for you two idiots, but y'all are trying my patience."

In my mind, my safety didn't really matter anymore. If I'd have stayed in Amarillo, I'd be dead anyway. Whatever happened now—running out of gas, stranded on a highway in the middle of nowhere, ending up on the evening news—it didn't matter. This was the resurrection tour. I might as well enjoy the ride.

We stayed that night at a nearby Motel 6 and set off for the final leg of our trip to Aunt Terri's the next morning.

Chapter 14

Fleabag Motels and False Hopes

W e drove nine hours the next day to make it to Bay St. Louis, Mississippi, a town about 33 miles west of Ocean Springs, Mississippi, where Aunt Terri lived. Instead of continuing on and showing up late, we decided it would be more polite to grab a motel and head to Terri's in the morning. That should have been the first hint of trouble on the horizon, but I totally missed it.

It wasn't until we pulled into the dumpy little motel parking lot that I knew we were in too deep. We were short on cash, out of moves, and still pretending everything was fine. All I could think was, "You've got to be kidding me." There we were, in Bay St. Louis, spending the night in a fleabag motel with nothing but $34 and half a tank of gas between the two of us. It was like we'd been treating the whole trip like we were on some divine mission from God…except the divine part hadn't shown up.

But wait—you haven't heard the kicker yet! *That's* when Mom finally called my Aunt Terri to let her know we were coming. Turns out, she hadn't called ahead like any person with common sense would. We'd just spent days driving from

Oklahoma City. And she only called Terri from the motel after we were practically already there.

I don't remember exactly what Mom said to Terri, but whatever she told her was total crap. It was at that moment that I realized that we weren't just winging it—we were lying, uninvited, and broke. I looked around the motel room, smelling mildew and God knows what else, thinking, *How the hell did I get here?*

Blues Brothers Energy

Aunt Terri said no.

Of course, Tanya had already called to warn Terri that we were coming, probably while we were still pulling out of Tanya's driveway. I'm sure she gave her the whole rundown.

"Hey, Aunt Terri, Shelly's on her way to see you. She's a mess, and Mom's with her. They packed up all their stuff in a U-Haul, and they're headed your way. Oh, and they've got Beau with them."

I guess if I were Terri, I might have said no too.

But that was it. Aunt Terri was our whole plan, and we had no backup. No place else to go. So what did we do?

With the gulf on one side and beachfront condos on the other, we drove down Highway 90 over and over and over for two straight days.

Were we desperate? Yes, but in a slaphappy, aimless kind of way. Think psychiatric hospital escapees with a dog and a U-Haul, and you've pretty much got the picture. Eventually, we realized how ridiculous we were being and started cracking jokes.

"Hey Mom, if anybody's sitting out on their condo balcony, they're sure getting an eyeful of us!"

She snickered. "They're probably wondering what the hell we're doing. The nosy old ladies are probably calling each other, saying, 'Hey Gladys! Guess what just went by on 90 again? That damn white car with the U-Haul! That's the third time today!'"

Those jokes would send us off into fits of laughter. Were we slightly unhinged, bordering on maybe-we've-completely-lost-it? I mean, yeah. We were hot. We were broke. We had a cocker spaniel in the backseat that was shedding like a cheap wig. I swear, if it hadn't been my real life, I'd have thought I was living a bad B movie plot.

The whole time, I kept thinking: *This is insane. This is completely insane.*

But it was still better than being back in Amarillo.

Chicken Drive-Thru Debacle

At one point during our Highway 90 purgatory loop, we decided we should eat something. So what do two exhausted, nearly broke women with a dog and a U-Haul do?

We went to look for a drive-thru. Naturally.

I think it was a chicken place—nothing fancy, just some fast food joint along the water. Neither of us wanted to leave Beau in the car alone—heaven forbid something happened to the dog—so we decided to try the drive-thru.

Great idea, right? It would have been…if we hadn't tried it with the whole damn rig, U-Haul and all.

About halfway through, one tire on the U-Haul caught the lip of a concrete retaining wall that blocked off a six-foot drop adjacent to the drive-thru lane. We accidentally drove that one wheel up onto the wall and almost tipped the trailer. If that trailer had tipped…truly, it still scares me to this day to think about it.

It took us over an hour to get out of that mess. The poor chicken place manager had to call someone to come help us. I don't even remember if we ended up with food. All I remember is the heat, the stress, and the absolute certainty that if we didn't die from embarrassment, we were definitely going to die from stupidity.

There we were, just two regular women trying to get some chicken, and we nearly flipped a trailer. I think that might have been the final straw for Aunt Terri.

By then, Mom had been calling her daily and giving her the updates on our insane Gulf Coast escapades. I'm sure she didn't tell her the *whole* truth, but Terri could tell things were unraveling. She just couldn't take it anymore. She was afraid we were going to end up dead or arrested. Neither of those options was ideal.

And so against all her better judgment and that of her Air Force husband, she let us come over.

A Temporary Landing

Once Aunt Terri finally caved and let us come, the only catch was the dog. She didn't want Beau in the house. And I get it. She already had two dogs—they were mutts, but she treated them like two expensive poodles with pedigrees. There was no way she was letting our show-quality cocker spaniel crash her mutt mansion.

We finally found a temporary place for Beau in Bay St. Louis that would board him for $25 a week with only a $15 deposit. They must've really been able to sense we were coming back for him, and, of course, we did.

We got Beau squared away and drove to Terri's, where we stayed for about ten days.

It wasn't long, but it was enough to catch our breath. It was nice to not have to live out of a U-Haul, wondering when the next gas station or chicken joint disaster was going to hit. We didn't belong there, and we knew we couldn't stay forever, but it was safe and quiet.

We took that little pocket of time to decide what we were going to do next. In a full-circle moment, we decided to head back to Texas and do what I'd wanted to do from the moment I'd taken myself out of high school. I was moving to Denton, a suburb of Dallas, to attend North Texas State University.

Chapter 15

College, Here I Come...or Not

M om and I had just lived through a whirlwind summer. We'd nearly run out of gas in Louisiana and slept in fleabag motels. We'd driven up and down Highway 90 for at least two straight days and got stuck on a drive-thru retaining wall at a chicken restaurant. We convinced my aunt to let us stay at her house, masked as a visit. And after all that craziness, Mom and I ended up heading to Denton, Texas.

Denton was a city just four hours from Amarillo. It was near Dallas, a major city, which seemed like a big step up for me. Nobody else seemed to think it was a good idea, though. Everybody—my dad, my grandmother, my sister—thought the Dallas area was too big and too dangerous for me. This time, though, Mom was okay with it, and I wasn't going to be denied. I had always wanted to live in Dallas. Once again, we loaded up the U-Haul and Beau and hit the road. We were going to Denton, where I'd enroll at North Texas State University. That was as far as our plan got, but it was better than no plan.

Of course, we rolled into Denton with nothing figured out. We had no idea where we'd live or what steps I'd need to take to enroll. We decided to take it one step at a time, and the first step was to get our hands on my GED certificate, which was back at the house. I couldn't set foot in Amarillo, so my mom dropped me off at another Motel 6 for the night, alone, and made the four-hour drive.

When she got to the house, she didn't stay long. She grabbed our stuff, my GED certificate, and some money. Then she closed up the house and dropped the U-Haul off at my grandmother's house so she could return it later. As she turned around and drove right back to Denton, I decided it was time to break the news to my dad that his little girl was moving to the big city.

Dad's idea was that I should stay local and go to Abilene Christian College or Clarendon Community College. But I knew his plan wasn't for me. I didn't want to move somewhere even smaller than Amarillo, and of course, staying in Amarillo was out of the question. Dad didn't have any idea why. He didn't even know I'd left town. It was time for me to call him to catch up.

"Hey, Dad."

"Hey, Shotgun," he answered. "So, I heard you left town."

"Yeah. I spent time at Tanya's and Aunt Terri's for a while. "

"Right. Well, where are you right now? What are your plans? Are you still in Mississippi?"

"No. I'm going to go to North Texas State."

He was silent for a moment, then, "Well, how do you plan on getting in there?"

"I'm in Denton now, enrolling," I said. Dad wasn't changing my mind this time, and I think he could hear the determination in my voice.

"Okay, well, let me know how it goes," he replied with a note of resignation in his voice. "Let me know what your plan is, and I'll see if I can help."

That was kind of how my dad was. I knew he loved me, but he was detached and uninvolved. If you were doing what he wanted you to do, he'd help. If not, maybe he wouldn't.

I still try to put myself in his shoes when I think about this situation sometimes, but I struggle to understand his perspective. After all, if your 17-year-old daughter suddenly left town and no one seemed to know where she'd gone or what had happened to her, wouldn't you be concerned? I would have been frantic if one of my boys suddenly disappeared off the face of the earth. But not my dad. As far as I know, even when I was "missing," he wasn't sending out flares to try to find me.

So I just kept doing what I always did—basically figuring out life on my own.

Enrolling at NTSU

The next morning, we were the first ones in line at the registrar's office at NTSU.

"Hi, I'm Shelly Grimm, and I'd like to enroll," I said. I'd never had any trouble letting people know what I wanted. "What do I need to do?"

The registrar looked at me, then reached into the filing cabinet next to her desk. "You'll need to submit these documents," she said, handing me a photocopied list of requirements for admission.

My stomach sank as I read through the list. We were totally unprepared. I don't think there was a single thing we could check off that list except for the GED certificate. After all, we hadn't really planned ahead for me to be going to college. I wasn't even supposed to be graduating from high school for another year. As usual, we were figuring things out as we went along.

Although we had my GED certificate, I needed my high school transcripts in order to register. I looked at Mom and knew she was going to have to get right back in the car and drive to Amarillo to get them.

Before we left, the woman at the registrar's office informed me I'd also need to take the ACT test. I was in luck, though, because they were offering it the next day. All we had to do was pay the testing fee and show up. The university called Dad, and to his credit, he paid the fee. I don't remember exactly how much the fee was, but no matter the amount, it was money we didn't have.

So, off Mom went to Amarillo to get my high school transcripts while I took the ACT. Within a couple of days, the results were in. I passed! I got the all clear from admissions, and I was officially a college student. Now all I had to do was register for classes and find a place to live.

A New Beginning

I'll never forget how it felt to stand in line to register for classes. I held a check from my dad for $128, enough to cover a full 12-hour load for the upcoming semester. That check felt like my golden ticket, and I couldn't wait to get started.

I also started looking for housing. Because the fall term was starting soon, the dorms were already full, and so were all the nearby one-bedroom apartments. The only thing I could find was a two-bedroom apartment off-campus, so I took it. Of course, my mom saw the open bedroom and took it as a sign.

"Well, maybe I'll come and live with you!"

Thankfully, once I was enrolled in college and moved into my new apartment, my mom went back to Amarillo—at least for a little while.

I loved college life. I really did. I had a schedule. I had a place of my own. I had some control. For once, I wasn't just reacting—I was actually *living*.

I picked forensic psychology as my major and sociology as my minor. NTSU ranked third in the country for its music school, so I also joined the choir. I found a job as a personal trainer at a club called National Health Studios, a large nationwide chain. This place was legit—even Dallas Cowboys football players worked out there.

That health club job brought me more than just a paycheck. It brought me my first new friend! She was a client who was probably around 25 or 26. We really hit it off during her training sessions, so on my days off, we'd hang out, sit in the hot tub, and talk.

There was no chaos in my life, and for the first time, I felt like I was where I was supposed to be. I was studying something that fascinated me. I had a little job, a little freedom, and a friend. And for that brief moment, I could breathe.

Beauty Queen and a Red Flag

Somewhere in the middle of getting ready for school and working at the health club, I won a beauty pageant.

You read that right—a freaking beauty pageant. I hadn't done a beauty pageant since I was a little kid, and I didn't really have any desire to do one in college. So you could say I wasn't very impressed when my mom walked into my new apartment one afternoon and announced that she'd signed me up for one.

"Come on, Shelly!" She could tell she was going to have to work hard to convince me to give it a shot. "It's a great way to get yourself out there and meet some people."

"I don't need to meet people. I already have a new friend."

"But you'll be so good at it! I already signed you up, so it's all settled."

"Okay, fine. But I may or may not do it," I warned her. Inside, I was fuming. How could she do something like that without even asking me? Then again, we're talking about my mom here. Tina did what Tina wanted, and apparently, Tina wanted to enter me in a beauty pageant. My new friend was there at the apartment with me when Mom told me, and she was no help. She just egged me on to do it too!

The pageant took place right before classes started that fall, and it was a big deal in Denton. Girls who'd been competing every year showed up in full pageant mode. They hired pageant coaches and invested in beautiful gowns with sequins and rhinestones. And me? I didn't even want to do it, but I did it anyway. I wore a bridesmaid's dress I had from my friend Cindy's wedding, the girl who lived on Clifton with me, and called it good. And you know what? I WON!

To be honest, I think I won because I didn't act like a teenager. I was seventeen, but I'd already lived through more than most of those girls ever would. That, and when they asked me, "What do you want to be?" I said, "I'm enrolled at North Texas State University, majoring in forensic psychology. I'm going to be a part of the Behavioral Analysis Unit." I think it was that answer that clinched the win. Most of the other contestants said, "I want to be a teacher" or "I'm going to beauty school." I gave the judges a unique answer and came across as a young woman with a plan. For the first time, I kind of was.

My winning the pageant caused a bit of a stir in more ways than one. I was the new girl, the underdog. All the repeat competitors and their mamas who had invested years of their lives and thousands of dollars in clothes, shoes, and pageant coaches were not impressed that some small-town girl from Amarillo had come in and swept the pageant. Pageant coaches took notice too. I got asked to work with the two top pageant coaches in the industry. They approached me, convinced I could win the Miss Texas pageant with their help.

Someone else took notice, too, but not in a good way. I'd kept in contact with my boyfriend, Jimmy, as well as I could over the summer, and our relationship was still going. But he wasn't so impressed with my pageant win. I was young, impressionable, and without parental support. Now, for the first time, he saw me doing something on my own that had nothing to do with him. I had a mother who was back in the picture, friends, a job, a pageant win, and a college life. My life was no longer orbiting around his choices of what he wanted, and he didn't like that. I think it scared him, and he wasn't about to let his prize (me) slip away. I'm not positive, but I think he thought he had me under his thumb.

So what did he do? He started flying me out to New Orleans to visit him every other weekend. I'd leave on Friday afternoons and fly back on Sunday nights. I felt really special and grown up at first. I had a hunky boyfriend paying for my airline tickets and taking me all over a fancy city every other weekend. What almost 18-year-old wouldn't love that?

Jimmy was a bartender, so when I went to visit him, I went to work with him. I'd help him get the bar ready and even sing with a few of the bands. We had a great time going from one bar to another. We partied all weekend long, then I'd hop on the flight back to Denton and sleep the whole way back. By the time my plane touched the ground, I was ready to spend the week as a college student again.

This went on for several months before reality set in. Paying for all those flights started getting expensive. He saw that I loved my weekends with him, and he was ready to move on to the next part of his plan. That's when he started asking me to move to New Orleans.

"Come on, Shelly," he'd try to persuade me. "We'll get married, and you can go to Tulane."

Honestly, it was flattering at first. He knew just what to say to make me feel like all my dreams were coming true. I had someone who loved me. Somebody who was going to take care of *me* for once.

I didn't know that things on his end were simmering below the surface, just waiting to explode and burst my happy bubble.

Leaving Denton, Again

In the end, it was a multitude of factors that pushed me out of Denton.

For one thing, partying all weekend and studying all week was starting to take its toll on me. Trying to keep all the plates in the air was stressing me out. And you know what else was stressing me out? My mom.

Yep, Mom had come back and made good on her word to move in with me. Now I was juggling school, an out-of-state boyfriend who wanted all of my time and attention, and a chronically ill mother who wanted the same. Maybe you remember the story at the beginning of the book where my mom was convinced I was bipolar and made me spend a week at the psychiatric hospital for blood tests. I don't know why, but it never occurred to her that maybe some of my stress could be attributed to her.

New Orleans started to sound more and more appealing. The test proved I wasn't bipolar—which wasn't a surprise to me—but something had to give or I really was going to lose it. In the end, it was another chronic illness that became the linchpin for my next stage of life.

My grandmother's cancer had come back, and this time, it had metastasized. As much as I had enjoyed having my apartment to myself before Mom had made good on her promise to move in with me, this wasn't my idea of a happy turn of events. My mom decided to go back to Amarillo to help, and I decided to withdraw from NTSU and move to New Orleans to be with Jimmy. Once again, the boxes came out, and the chaos kicked back in.

We packed up everything—my mom's stuff and mine. In what felt like a massive case of déjà vu, we loaded all her and Beau's stuff into a U-Haul. I packed what I could into two blue Samsonite suitcases and an overnight bag.

We hugged goodbye in the parking lot of the apartment complex, then we each got in our separate rides and drove in opposite directions at the same time. She took Beau and the U-Haul and headed back to Amarillo. And my fitness client-turned-friend drove me to the airport.

That was the last time I ever lived in Denton.

It wouldn't be long before I started wishing I had never left.

When the Switch Flipped

New Orleans was supposed to be exactly like the weekends we'd spent together. That's the way Jimmy sold it to me, anyway. Those weekends were a great time, so of course I had no problem moving there. We'd just keep enjoying the jazz, crawfish boils, and late nights. It felt like a movie—the kind where everything finally goes right in the end.

But the feeling didn't last.

You know the old story about the man faced with the decision between going to Heaven or going to Hell when he dies? In the joke, the man is given the opportunity to preview both Heaven and Hell before he chooses which place he would like to spend eternity. He decides to preview Hell first.

When he gets there, the devil, a handsome, charming fellow, shows him the sights. He even points out all his old friends, who are having the time of their lives doing nothing but golfing, drinking, and having fun. He and the devil chit chat like old buddies, and before he leaves, the devil gives him a brochure that details everything they had seen.

Next, the man previews Heaven, where Saint Peter meets him at the gate. In Heaven, the man sees family and loved ones who have passed on before him. They are all very sweet and kind. Everything is beautiful. The streets are paved with gold, and the weather is perfect, but compared to hell, where his golf buddies were, it seems pretty boring.

The man decides that Hell is definitely where he wants to go.

When the man dies the next day, however, his experience is much different. He's greeted at the gates of Hell by an ugly, despicable monster. "Who are you?" the man asks in horror.

"Don't you recognize me, old buddy? It's me, the devil," he says with an evil grin. "Now, let's get you settled."

The devil ushers the man through the fire and brimstone. People are screaming in agony; it's sweltering in there, and all of the people are chained and dragging their chains around.

There are no golf courses, no drinking buddies. None of what the man saw the day before seems to even exist in this place! He doesn't understand—this is not the future he'd been shown. It was like a switch had been flipped.

"Hey, what happened?" he asked the devil with panic in his voice. "This isn't what I saw yesterday!" He tries to pull the brochure the devil had given him out of his pocket as proof, but it disintegrates in his hand.

"Oh, that? Yesterday, I was just campaigning," the devil said with a sneer. "Today, I'm in office."

That's what happened to me when I moved to New Orleans. It was like a switch flipped, and a whole lot of stuff that hadn't been in the "brochure" started coming to light. Within the first week, Jimmy got fired, and somehow, it was my fault. And since I was the reason he lost his job, I had to find a full-time job. He was a master at twisting things around and making me feel like I was to blame for everything.

I started to see through the lies and control Jimmy kept me under. But still, I stayed. I didn't have anywhere else to go. He had me, period. The charm, the attention, the flights—it was all part of his "campaign." Once I moved to New Orleans and got unpacked, it was like he owned me. I'd been sold a dream that didn't exist, and none of what was happening to me had been in the preview. Instead of enrolling at Tulane and finishing my degree, I went to work at Village Lady in Lake Forest Mall.

It still astounds me how quickly the switch flipped. One minute I was singing in the bar and laughing until the sun came up. Next, I was crying on the phone to my mom every day for two years straight.

This wasn't what I'd signed up for, but it was what I had. And I was going to spend the next few years paying the price. I thought I'd be getting freedom, but instead I just had another person to take care of.

And it was going to get much worse before it got better.

CONCLUSION

When you're walking through the fire of chronic illness—whether it's your own or someone else's—there's no manual. No perfect roadmap. Survival often hinges on a person's ability to adapt, ask for help, and push forward regardless of the circumstances. A healthy sense of humor doesn't hurt either!

But survival can also hinge on others' willingness to pay attention to the signs that you need help and reach out to offer that help. My story reveals the cracks in the systems that weren't even an afterthought, but would have been there to protect me, and I've done my best to point toward what *could* be done differently so that others who find themselves in similar situations can be better supported than I was.

People, especially caregivers who are still children, need real support, a listening ear, and serious follow-through from people around them who care. Don't let my story be just a cautionary tale that you read and then put on a shelf. Let this story be your call to action to pay attention to the people around you and speak up when you see a child in need.

Doing Things Differently

You may have noticed that the chapters in part 3 of this book don't have the "Doing Things Differently" section at the end.

That was intentional. These chapters mark the beginning of my adulthood, where I was finally old enough that it was reasonable for me to make the decisions I'd *already* been making for years. I was at the point where there had been no one looking out for me for so long that I assumed what I was dealing with was normal. I didn't recognize unhealthy patterns. The lessons hadn't settled yet, and I hadn't come out the other side. Sometimes you don't get the clarity until much, much later. Sometimes, you don't get it at all until you're ready to tell the story out loud. That's where I was then. Still learning. Still just trying to survive.

I built my whole career around making sure families are financially prepared for chronic illness because I know what happens when they're not. After everything I went through with my mom and then again with my son, I realized nobody was coming to save us. That's why I learned how to help others get the right insurance products in place *before* their lives fall apart.

This book is for all the caregivers who are hurting. You're not alone. The Perpetual Caregiver Collective is here to help. The Perpetual Caregiver Collective is a group of passionate, caring professionals in a variety of fields who provide resources, retreats, or respite to restore your mind, body, and soul. For more information about this collective, visit www. ThePerpetualCaregiver.com/collective.

Thank you for joining me on my journey as my mother's caregiver. I hope this book has given you tools you can use to help you through your journey, whether you're a caregiver or someone living with a chronic illness. Although this is the end of *Some Asses Just Need Wiping*, this isn't the end of my story. The next 14 years were some of the most devastating and brutal in my life. And also where I fell in love with the city of New Orleans and learned some of the most important lessons that eventually helped me figure out exactly where I fit into the world. To discover what happened after I moved to New Orleans, married Jimmy, and became a caregiver for another chronic illness sufferer, be on the lookout for my next book, *Some Loves Just Need Leaving*.

ACKNOWLEDGEMENTS

I want to extend my heartfelt thanks to all those who supported me during the writing of this book. My love, compassion, and devotion go out to my mother, who was the original catalyst for *Some Asses Just Need Wiping*. Through the process of writing, I truly came to realize the profound struggles she faced. Her courage, fierce nature, and tenacity in the face of impossible odds have inspired me and are woven into this work, as well as the initiative, The Perpetual Careviger Collective.

It is crucial to acknowledge that no one, including the medical community, truly understood what we were dealing with at the time. In light of this, I extend grace to all of us for the challenges we faced together.

I also want to express my gratitude to my love and soulmate, Kris, who stood by me through every late night and countless revisions. Your unwavering support and belief in me provided the strength to bring this project to fruition. I am incredibly thankful to my marketing and launch team for their creativity and dedication in bringing this book to life, and to my editor, Christa, for her keen eye and thoughtful suggestions that shaped this manuscript.

Thank you all for being part of this journey; your support means the world to me.

PERPETUAL CAREGIVER RESOURCES

You can now visit theperpetualcaregiver.com — a space created specifically for caregivers and those who love them. This isn't just a site; it's a gathering place for real talk, real tools, and real encouragement. You'll find:

- Stories that speak the caregiver's truth
- Updates on my book and events
- Access to the powerful Family Love Letter tool
- Invitations to connect, learn, and laugh a little

If you're new to being a family caregiver, here are some tips that can help you navigate the unique challenges that come with caregiving.[5]

Tips for Family Caregivers

As I was beginning to prepare this section, my phone rang. It was the husband of one of my very closest friends, Tracy. Tracy is someone who has been in my corner since we were

---

5   Melinda Smith, M.A., Jeanne Segal, Ph.D., and Lawrence Robinson, "Family Caregiving," *HelpGuide*, last updated January 16, 2025, https://www.helpguide.org/family/caregiving/family-caregiving

teenagers. I'd even consider her a member of my own care team, although I didn't know what a care team was back then.

Remember that rager of all ragers at my house in the spring before I left Amarillo? The morning after the party, Tracy came over to my house, woke me up around 7:00 a.m., and took me up to the grocery store, where we bought all kinds of cleaning supplies. Then we came back to my house, and she helped me clean it from stem to stern.

This same friend suffered a massive stroke three years ago, and it hit me hard. This phone call brought more bad news. Tracy had been admitted to the hospital for another possible stroke. She was stable, but they were awaiting results from some of the tests, so they knew what they were really dealing with.

I began to realize that I could publish 100 pages of tips, hacks, advice, websites, and 1-800 numbers and gather up the information for every association under the sun, and it would still fall short. All of that information still fails to adequately prepare a person for the road ahead with their loved ones. Each situation is so individual and unique because there are different personalities and human beings involved.

Don't give up. There are options and resources available to you. For me, I know God is what got me through every single moment of my childhood. I had no idea at the time what to do or who to talk to. As I mentioned in the book, there was no one to lean on because no one was making themselves readily available. I didn't have any siblings living with me, and my mother was ill. So when I was by myself, I played church. I sat my stuffed animals and dolls all over my room, and I preached. And boy did I preach!

As for where to start your search for resources to get you and your loved one through this season, I recommend that you start with prayer. One knee is good, but two knees are better.

Then, start reaching out to any group or person who has offered to help in the past or who even remotely sounds like they might be able to help you. Believe me, someone will get you on the road to the right people—but you must stay diligent. There are so many resources available, so don't give up.

Write things down. Keep diligent notes. Record the names and contact information for each person you speak with. You'll be glad you did. When I was finally able to have agency over my situation, I kept an entire notebook dedicated just to my mother.

You are your loved ones' advocate. They may not be able to be their own advocate at this time or maybe ever, so if you're not used to advocating for someone else, this might be something you'll need to practice. Don't be afraid to make waves or speak up if you have questions or concerns. It's important that you understand what is happening too.

Study and research everything you can, including their condition and the options for treatment and care. The more you know, the better you will be able to handle issues as they come up.

And take time for yourself. If your loved one or family member has health insurance or is on a government-funded insurance plan, they may have respite coverage in their policy. If so, you can use that to recharge occasionally so that you can manage all that comes with the role of caregiver, whether it be paid or unpaid.

I tell ya, I have so many ideas, I should write another book! Oh, wait a minute—I am! I look forward to sharing the next chapter with you. We'll see each other soon. Take good care until then.

Shelly

ABOUT THE AUTHOR

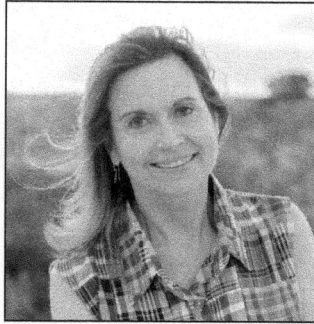

S **helly Grimm** is the author of *Some Assess Just Need Wiping*, her debut memoir that explores the impact of chronic illness on families and relationships through the lens of her own caregiving journey. A financial services professional with 27 years of experience, she brings unique insight into the importance of support systems and financial preparedness, having grown up without access to such coverage. Through her work with her organization, The Perpetual Caregiver, Shelly aims to empower everyone, including caregivers, to gain knowledge and find strength, resilience, and the resources they need along the way to avoid the pitfalls that can occur without those missing pieces.